PLANT BASED DIET MEAL PLAN

Easy And Healthy Plant Based Recipes For Everyone

CAROLINE EMILIA LAW

Text Copyright © [CAROLINE EMILIA LAW]

Legal & Disclaimer

The information contained in this book and its contents is not designed to replace or take the place of any form of medical or professional advice; and is not meant to replace the need for independent medical, financial, legal or other professional advice or services, as may be required. The content and information in this book has been provided for educational and entertainment purposes only.

The content and information contained in this book has been compiled from sources deemed reliable, and it is accurate to the best of the Author's knowledge, information and belief. However, the Author cannot guarantee its accuracy and validity and cannot be held liable for any errors and/or omissions. Further, changes are periodically made to this book as and when needed. Where appropriate and/or necessary, you must consult a professional (including but not limited to your doctor, attorney, financial advisor or such other professional advisor) before using any of the suggested remedies, techniques, or information in this book.

Upon using the contents and information contained in this book, you agree to hold harmless the Author from and against any damages, costs, and expenses, including any legal fees potentially resulting from the application of any of the information provided by this book. This disclaimer applies to any loss, damages or injury caused by the use and application, whether directly or indirectly, of any advice or information presented, whether for breach of contract, tort, negligence, personal injury, criminal intent, or under any other cause of action.

You agree to accept all risks of using the information presented inside this book.

You agree that by continuing to read this book, where appropriate and/or necessary, you shall consult a professional (including but not limited to your doctor, attorney, or financial advisor or such other advisor as needed) before using any of the suggested remedies, techniques, or information in this book.

Table of Contents

INTRODUCTION

Many people have taken lightly about eating healthy diet. Most thinks that healthy foods are too much of a hassle to make, takes a very long time to cook and the ingredients are hard to be found in the supermarkets near them. All of these excuses seem silly and whatnot, but the sad part is that many people are choosing to be ignorant about making their lifestyle better, even though they know that it is for their own good in the long run.

It is normal to see people following the trend of eating urban foods or participating in food challenge without knowing why they do it and what the consequences are. For examples, currently, there is a so called *"boba* milk tea" wave happening in Southeast Asia and many people are willing to pay such an unhealthy drink which contain at least 16 tablespoons of sugars every day at different outlets just for getting Instagram likes without thinking about the consequences to their health. These *boba* milk teas is originated from Taiwan, which originally consists of milk tea and tapioca balls (*boba*) cooked in a large amount of melted brown sugar. What is more concerning is that people who are participating in this trend are younger people who are supposedly aware of the consequences beforehand by asking experts or doing some research?

Encouraging people to eat healthy have long been done by organizations, but people still choosing to eat oily and fast foods that are high in calorie. These types of foods are commonly quicker to make and tasty as well, making them the favorite choice of foods. Furthermore, healthy diet should not only start when one has just beginning to go to the gym and exercise regularly, but it should be instilled in our mind since we were at a young age that healthy diet is an important aspect of life as we are going to be using our body systems regularly. Parents should have learnt their lesson and educate their children from home about healthy diet or living healthy as they have more access to their children than any other person.

Another important point about healthy diet is that it is just not good enough to eat healthy alone without physical exercises. Many people think that they are healthy enough just because they follow healthy diet plan. However, this is half true because healthy diet could improve your health, but exercising could optimize your health performance further. People who have the desire to lose weight especially, are encouraged to do physical exercises or workouts at least 3-4 times a week for about an hour for an optimal result. This should come along with healthy food consumption. One thing you should avoid in healthy dieting is that you should not eat oily food for post workouts /exercises because you will on regain the calories after burning about hundreds of them at the gym. This will leave a very minimum impact to your body. Stay consistent with healthy diet especially with the amount of food intake even if it is on your cheat day!

My only hope for my readers is to make them realize how easy it is to cook plant-based foods and that I hope everyone could benefit from the recipes and health facts in this book. Happy reading!

PART I: WHAT IS PLANT-BASED DIET?

When you hear about plant-based diet, you would think that it is expensive, tasteless and sometimes bitter, because of its plant-based ingredients. Well, this is truly a myth that has been injected into our minds since we were a child, not to mention that we dislike the taste of any vegetables that are served for us. It is time to change that mindset of ours to be more accepting of plant-based diet and accept the fact that it is greatly beneficial for our body and mind.

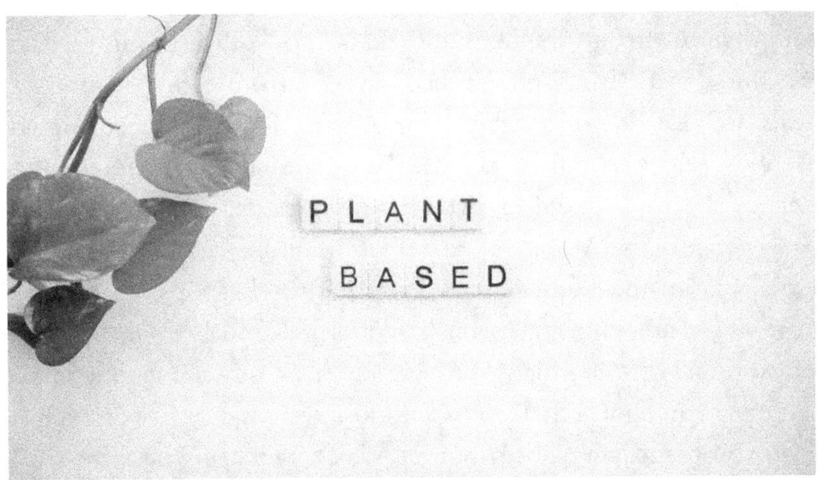

Basically, a plant-based diet consists of plant-based ingredients including vegetables, fruits, whole grains, legumes, seeds, and nuts, and that unhealthy ingredients such as sugars and refined grains are eliminated. From those lists, some of you might be questioning where the source of proteins would come from if we only eat these foods all the time. Now this is another myth that should be clarified. Proteins found in plants such as soy, soluble fibres (oats and barley) and almonds are as good as those found in fish and meats. Those who practice a plant-based diet are restricted to not consume meat, poultry, fish, milk, eggs, honey or animal-based products, or processed vegan foods. This diet is all about eating clean, meaning eating simple and whole foods. Moreover, you would get more insight into what each ingredient in a plant-based meal does to your body.

The most important thing about plant-based diet is that, it is useful if you are planning to lose some weight and get into a better shape other than doing exercises. From the book entitled "The Greenprint" by Marco Borges, an acquaintance of his managed to drop his weight for 200 pounds in about over two-and-a-half years ever since he started to practice eating plant-based foods, apart from doing some work outs for five to six times a week. Not only that, in this case, the first thing that Mr. Borges' friend noticed from eating plant-based meals are that he got a lighter complexion, felt more energetic and his body felt lighter than before. These are some of the common changes that you would experience after practicing plant-based diet for several years. Moreover, a research finding conducted by Dr Bernard from the Physician's Committee for Responsible Medicine suggested that practicing plant-based diet is much easier than the conventional diet at which you have to check on your calorie intake. These evident shows that you would lose weight even if you eat a lot when you practice a plant-based diet. Isn't it amazing how the foods that you eat could lead to a bigger effect to your body?

Plant-based diet could provide many benefits to your body and mind. It has been associated with many health benefits such as reducing risks of heart diseases, depression, dementia, diabetes, and obesity. This fact is further supported by the findings presented during the Vegetarian Congress in 2013 that continuously suggested plant-based eaters have lower blood cholesterol levels, blood sugars, and blood pressure compared to meat eaters as these factors are the symptoms of heart disease and cancer. Generally, plant-based diet is connected to fiber-rich foods due to its nature of containing fiber that could help in constipation and digestion, and many other health benefits. In this part, I will list out some of the common health benefits that you would get by eating plant-based diet.

A good starter for weight-loss

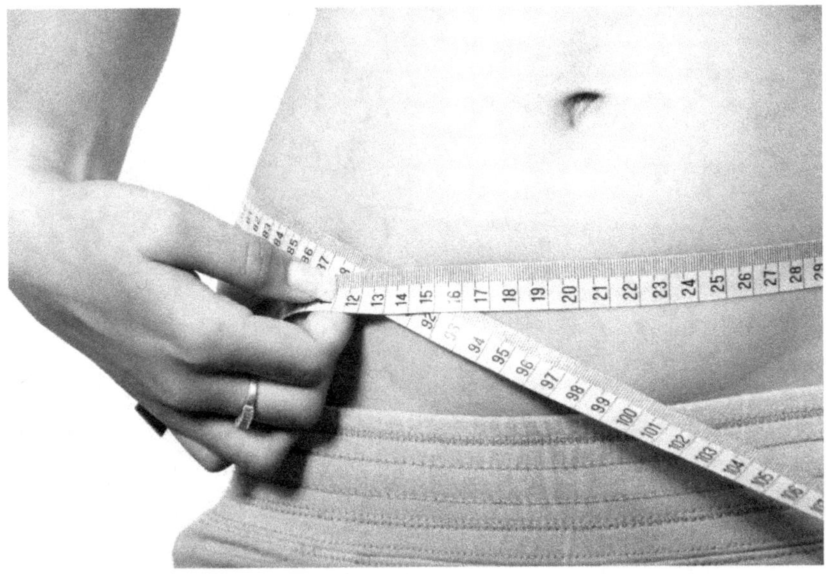

Consuming plant-based diet means that you are eliminating meat, dairy or processed food from your body system by not consuming them. These foods contain unhealthy fats which are bad for your body and could affect your system if taken in a large amount or frequently.

Good for detoxifying your body

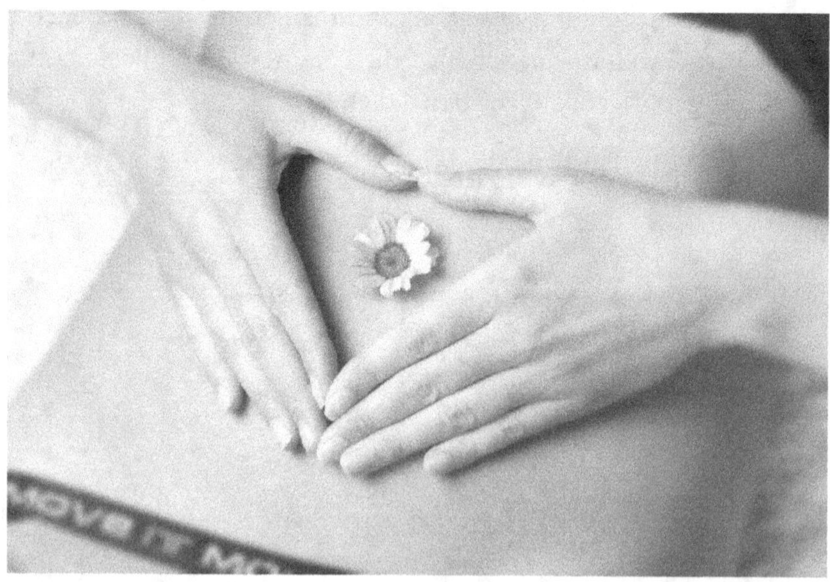

As you consume more plant-based food, you will soon realize that your body is starting to become naturally cleaner and lighter than before, and that you will get a lighter complexion too around your face. This is good news for women in particular to have a better skin naturally. Plant-based diet are said to be able to detoxify your body because with this diet, you will consume less chemicals, pesticides, hormones and antibiotics which are typically found in animal-based products or foods. Other than that, high-fiber citrusy fruits such as apples, raspberries, blueberries and oranges are also commonly known to supply a good amount of vitamin C to the body and said to be good detoxifying agents.

Reducing risk of heart diseases

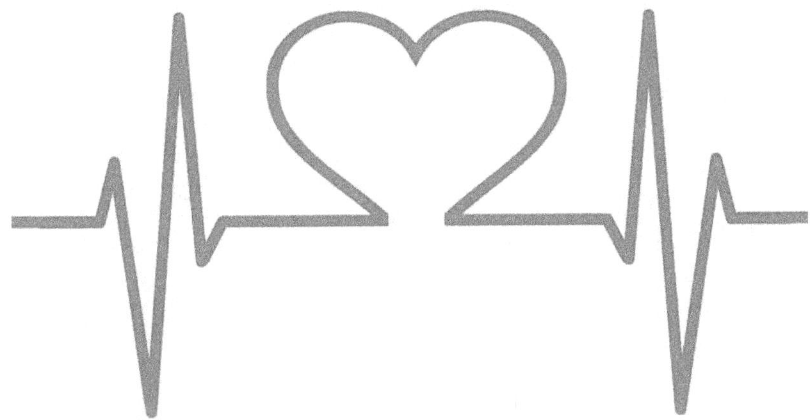

Which is one of the many diseases that killed millions of people all around the world? As you consume more plant-based foods, you are actually reducing the risk of having heart diseases or any diseases that might block your artery system which originated from unsaturated animal fats. On the other hand, healthy unsaturated fats such as avocados, seeds, nuts, legumes and wheat could decrease your cholesterol and fatty layer levels.

Improve your vision

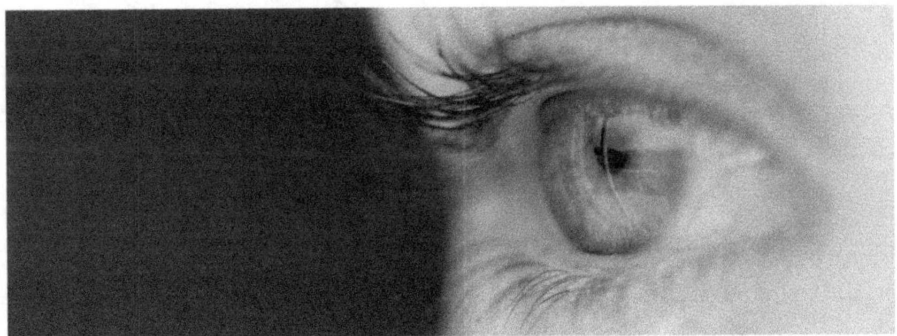

Apart from the common health benefits that plant-based diet could offer, this diet plan could also improve your night vision in particular. Plant-based sources such as spinach, carrot, kale, corn, kiwi and squash are rich in lutein and zeaxanthin pigments which could prevent cataract and macular degeneration. Macular degeneration is typically found in older people aged 60 and above, whereby their visions are not able to function well, and they may have lost their sight irreversibly.

Good for constipation and digestion

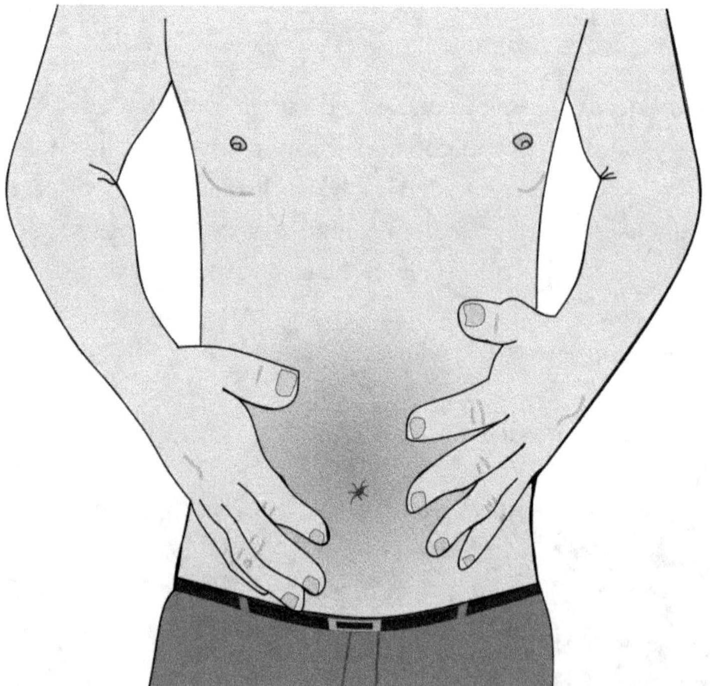

Plant-based diet consists of sources that are rich in fibers and could lower your blood sugar and cholesterol levels. According to the Medical News Today portal, legumes such as beans, lentils and peas contains high amount of fibers and that they are good to lower the rate of type 2-diabetes and obesity. Furthermore, green vegetables and fruits are a good source of fiber to prevent constipation and improve digestion which in turns leading to easier weight loss compared to just cutting down your calorie intake. A good bowel could prevent cancer which could affect the digestive system such as colon cancer as holding your waste in would only increase the risk of having this type of cancer.

PART II: PLANT-BASED DIET MEAL PLAN

I have designed a plant-based diet meal plan suitable for newcomers, especially those who are planning to change their eating habit. Not only that, individuals who would like to try new ideas into their plant-based diet meal plan or daily cooking could also try the recipes in which I will include in the next part of this book. The meals in this plan are for a duration of fourteen days which consist of breakfast, lunch, dinner, dessert and snack using ingredients which you can find easily and you may switch the turns as per your preference or even add new menus into the plan.

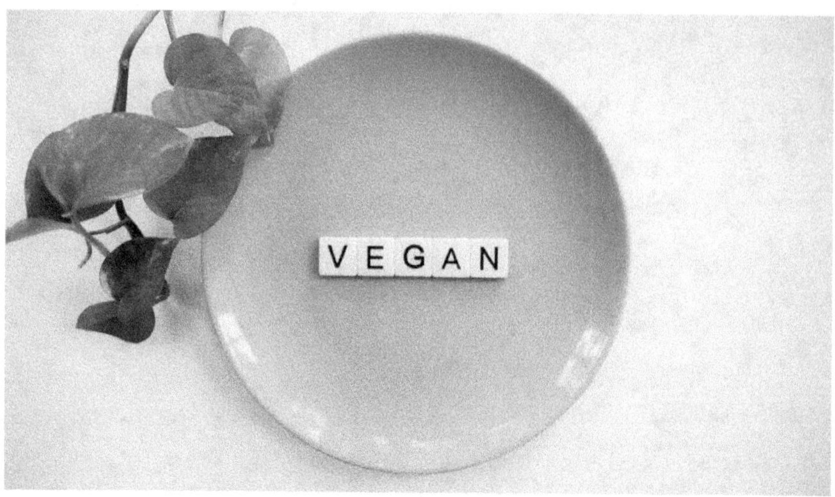

Menu	Day 1	Day 2
Breakfast	Banana pancake	Berry with ginger smoothie
Lunch	Stuffed bell peppers with tofu and zucchini	Spinach with strawberry salad
Snack	Chocolate covered banana ice cream bars	Miso soup
Dinner	Tomato with tofu soup	Vegetarian meatballs with spaghetti
Dessert	Grilled peaches	Vanilla ice cream

Menu	Day 3	Day 4
Breakfast	Fresh fruit salad	Potato waffles
Lunch	Mushroom and broccoli soup	Leek potato soup
Snack	Greek pasta salad	Winter vegetable salad
Dinner	Lentil Shepherd's pie	Creamy chowder with corn and fennel
Dessert	Chocolate peanut butter truffles	Chocolate orange mousse

Menu	Day 5	Day 6
Breakfast	Breakfast sandwiches with peanut butter and fresh fruits	Strawberry oatmeal breakfast smoothie

Lunch	Tasty greens with garlic	Farro lentil salad
Snack	Blood orange salad	Creamy spinach
Dinner	Chickpea noodle soup	Carrot soup with fresh ginger
Dessert	Coconut-banana cookie	Pumpkin pie

Menu	Day 7	Day 8
Breakfast	Chickpea omelette	Breakfast scramble
Lunch	Spiral pasta with tofu, zucchini and bell peppers	Creamy pumpkin soup
Snack	Potato salad	Carrot and shredded beet salad
Dinner	Shiitake mushroom with bean sprouts and chilli soup	Tofu kebabs with zucchini and eggplants
Dessert	Almond cheesecake	Lemon meringue pie

Menu	Day 9	Day 10
Breakfast	Peanut butter and raspberry jam porridge	Toast with avocado and scrambled tofu
Lunch	Zucchini noodles with portobello bolognese	Sweet and sour cauliflower with rice
Snack	Classic coleslaw	Corn salad

Dinner	Butternut squash soup with spices	Spinach soup with mint
Dessert	Apple pie	Chocolate-dipped fruits with spices
Menu	**Day 11**	**Day 12**
Breakfast	French toast with banana cream and blueberry	Roasted garlic potatoes
Lunch	Simple cauliflower rice	Mushroom, kale and barley pilaf
Snack	Plant sausages with rice salad	Sriracha almonds
Dinner	Korean style tofu	Spicy black beans with corn soup
Dessert	Mango and coconut sorbet	Fruity shave ice
Menu	**Day 13**	**Day 14**
Breakfast	Fruity banana split	Simple peanut butter breakfast bar
Lunch	Tofu tacos	Middle-eastern style plant-based pizza
Snack	Carrot salad	Crunchy silverbeet slaw
Dinner	Turmeric cauliflower	Spicy stir-fry tofu

Dessert	Black sesame soymilk-shake	Berry almond crisp

PART III: THE RECIPES

This part emphasizes on the recipe of the dishes of the plant-based diet meal plan in the previous part. These recipes are quick and easy to follow, with ingredients which can easily be found near you. For an optimum effect of this diet for your body, I suggest you to find fresh and organic ingredients if possible. Happy cooking!

BREAKFAST

Starting your day with all the necessary nutrients in your body is important to keep you energized throughout the day. The two most important nutrients that have to be included in your breakfast are carbohydrate and protein, which would guarantee a long-lasting energy. Below are the breakfast recipes as per included in the meal plan.

1. Banana pancake
2. Berry with ginger smoothie
3. Fresh fruit salad
4. Potato waffles
5. Breakfast sandwiches with peanut butter and fresh fruits
6. Strawberry oatmeal breakfast smoothie
7. Chickpea omelette
8. Breakfast scramble
9. Peanut butter with raspberry jam porridge
10. Toast with avocado and scrambled tofu
11. French Toast with Banana Cream and Blueberry
12. Roasted garlic potatoes
13. Fruity banana split
14. Simple peanut butter breakfast bar

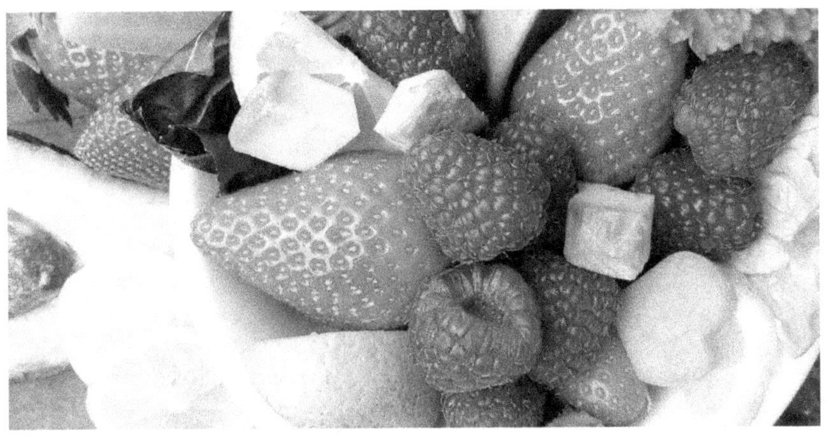

BANANA PANCAKE

Ingredients:

- 2 ripe bananas
- 1 cup rolled oats
- ¼-1/2 cups almond milk
- Organic maple syrup
- Cinnamon (optional; for dusting or more rich flavour)

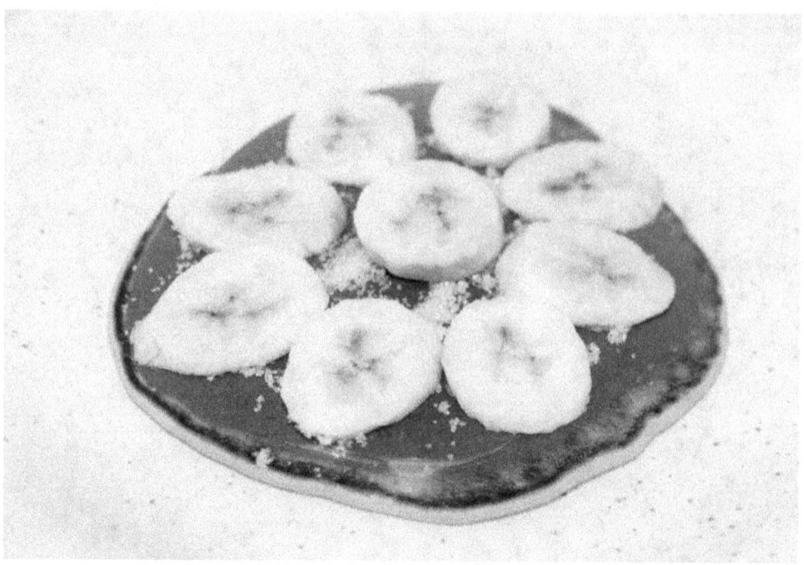

Methods:

1. Blend the bananas, rolled oats, cinnamon and almond milk until smooth (start with a small amount of milk then gradually increase until you get the typical pancake batter consistency).

2. Heat a pan with coconut oil over a low or medium heat.

3. Pour the batter on the hot pan until golden brown on both sides. For a practical method to pour your batter onto the pan, fill it in a small water jug or a ketchup bottle so you do not overpour the batter.

4. Cook on one side until there are bubbles appearing on the uncooked surface and until your spatula can firmly slide underneath it, then flip the cake.

5. Serve with an organic maple syrup for sweetness and enjoy your morning with a healthy and filling breakfast meal.

Health fact

✓ Apart from being good for dietary fibre such as preventing constipation, banana is rich in vitamin B6 and C, as well as cholesterol and sodium-free which are perfect for your diet and energy supply during the day.

✓ Organic maple syrup is an alternative to sugar and other sweetener agents which have plenty of health benefits, particularly the skin. These health benefits including its role as a good antioxidant, keeps our skin healthy, prevent cancer disease and have low Glycemic Index (GI) value, which is the ranking value for the carbohydrate or glucose contents in our food.

BERRY WITH GINGER SMOOTHIE

Ingredients:

- ½ cup frozen raspberries
- ½ cup strawberries
- ½ cup steamed cauliflower
- 1 one-inch cube ginger
- 1 cup almond milk (or any plant-based milk)
- 1 tbsp of chia seed (optional)
- Ice cubes (optional)

Methods:

1. Blend all of the ingredients until smooth.

2. You may add some chia seed to the blend if you like your smoothie to be thicker and richer.

3. If you prefer it cold, add some ice cubes into your glass but not too much! You don't want it to taste like plain water after some time.

4. Drink straight away and you're ready to start your day!

Health fact

✓ Berries provides plenty of fibres, thus good for the digestive system.

✓ Berries are relatively low in calorie; one cup of strawberries contains about 50 calories while one cup of raspberries contains about only 64 calories.

✓ Gingers are good to prevent many types of nausea such as the sea sickness, morning sickness and the after-surgery nausea.

✓ Gingers are also proven to be good source of cure for cold and flu.

FRESH FRUIT SALAD

Ingredients:

Dressing

- ½ raw soaked cashews

- ½ plant milk (soy milk, rice milk, etc.)

- 6 dates, pitted (for sweetness)

- ½ tsp vanilla

Fruits Salad

- ½ cup toasted and chopped walnuts

- 2 bananas, sliced

- 1 cup of fresh blackberries

- 1 cup of fresh kiwis

- 1 cup of fresh strawberries

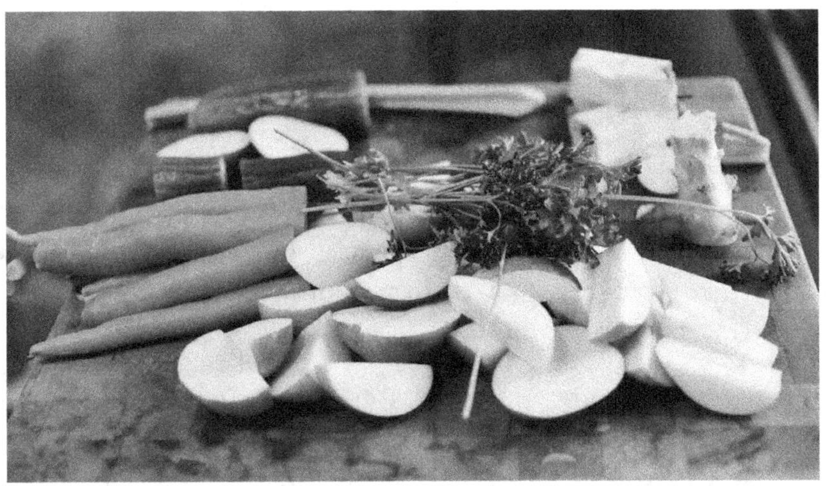

Methods:

For dressing:

1. Roast raw cashews until golden brown, and then chop into chunks for easy blending with the other ingredients.

2. Blend milk, dates, vanilla and roasted cashews until smooth.

3. Set aside for a while.

For salad:

1. Cut fresh kiwis and strawberries into medium chunks until they fill up one measuring cup respectively.

2. Put all fruits together into a salad bowl.

3. Pour the dressing and sprinkle some toasted walnuts on top.

4. Ready to be served.

Health fact:

✓ Soy milk is a good source of vitamin A, vitamin B, protein and potassium. It is also low in calorie compared to whole milk and have as much protein as cow's milk. This milk is also beneficial to lower the risk of cancer, osteoporosis and menopausal syndrome.

✓ Walnuts and cashews are both good source of fibre. However, the fibre content in walnuts are more than that in cashews. The fat most commonly found in nuts are mostly healthy unsaturated fat, however, they are also high in calories. Therefore, the intake of nuts in the daily diet should be taken in moderation.

✓ Eating fruits for breakfast is the best alternative since they are low in calorie and rich in health goodness. Besides that, you could also lower your blood sugar level by eating fruits because each fruit contain their own natural sugar.

POTATO WAFFLES

Ingredients:

- 4 medium-sized potatoes, unpeeled
- ½ cup soy milk (or any other plant milk of your choice)
- ½ cup of plain flour
- ¼ tsp garlic powder
- ¼ tsp paprika
- ¼ tsp nutmeg
- Salt
- Pepper

Methods:

1. Boil the potatoes until they are soft and easy to be mashed later on. Put aside for a while to leave it cool.

2. After a few minutes of cooling the potatoes, mash them then gradually add plain flour and milk until well combined.

3. Add plain flour, garlic powder, paprika, nutmeg salt and pepper into the mixture until well combined with medium consistency, not too runny and not too solid. You should expect the colour to be slightly yellowish or orange due to the paprika.

4. Spread your waffle maker with some corn oil or any other vegetarian oil before putting your batter into the maker.

Different waffle maker has different instructions, so follow yours accordingly before putting the batter.

5. Toast the waffles until golden brown and crispy on the outside.

6. Serve with maple syrups for sweetness or ketchup if you like it savoury, otherwise you can eat it plain.

Health fact

✓ Potato skins consist of plenty vitamins and minerals and that peeling them would lower the nutritional content of potatoes. However, since the method of cooking varies, thus the nutritional content would also vary. For example, fried potatoes contain more calorie than that of boiled or baked ones.

✓ Potatoes could also increase blood sugar control as it contains resistance starch which is not full broken down and absorbed by the body. It is also associated with type decreasing insulin resistance in type 2 diabetes which resulted in a better removal of the excess blood sugar.

BREAKFAST SANDWICHES WITH PEANUT BUTTER AND FRESH FRUITS

Ingredients:

- 2 slices of wholemeal bread

- 1 tbsp of unsweetened peanut butter

- 1 banana

- 1 strawberry

- 5 blueberries

Methods:

1. Spread peanut butter onto a slice bread evenly.

2. Cut the banana and strawberry into bitesize pieces and spread them on top of the peanut butter spread.

3. Put the other slice of bread on top and it is ready to be served.

   *best served with almond milk or coffee

<u>Health fact</u>

- ✓ Wholemeal bread is rich in fibre and could prevent bowel cancer and could assist with weight loss. Other than that, it is also packed with nutrients such as minerals, vitamin B and vitamin E.

✓ A study found that those who consume wholemeal bread tends to be slimmer since it could keep them full throughout the day.

✓ The daily recommendation of whole grain consumption per person is three servings or 48g per day, which is equivalent to two slices of wholemeal bread.

STRAWBERRY OATMEAL BREAKFAST SMOOTHIE

Ingredients:

- 1 cup plant-based milk (soy milk, almond milk, etc.).

- 2 cups frozen strawberries

- ½ cup rolled oats

- 1 tbsp maple syrup (optional)

- ½ tsp vanilla extract

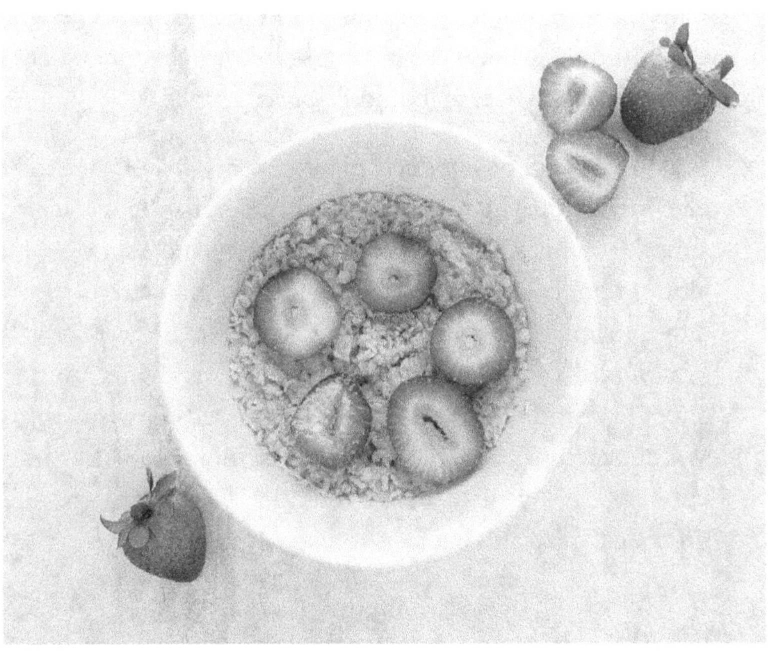

Methods:

1. Put the rolled oats into a blender or a food processor to slightly grind them up.

2. In the same blender or food processor, add the milk, strawberries, maple syrup and vanilla extract then blend them together until smooth.

3. Serve with ice cubes or you could also drink it straight away.

Health fact

✓ Just like wholemeal, oats could also keep you full all day and is generally good for metabolic health such as digestion.

✓ Oats is also found to be as good as taking hypertensive medication to lower blood pressure which could decrease cardiovascular disease in middle-aged people.

✓ It is hard to choose which plant-based milk are healthier as all of them provide plenty of health benefits. However, for a simple comparison between soymilk and almond milk, almond milk contains lower calorie compared to soymilk while soymilk contains higher protein than almond milk. See? It's very hard to choose which one is better, but that shouldn't stop you from using plant-based milk in your diet! Whichever it is, use the one that is most suitable for your cooking as any plant-based milk are guaranteed to offer a great deal of health benefits to us.

CHICKPEA OMELETTE

Ingredients:

Batter

- ¾ cups chickpea flour (grounded raw chickpea)

- ¾ cups plant-based milk (soy milk, almond milk, etc.)

- 2 tsp apple cider vinegar

- ¼ tsp turmeric powder

- ¼ tsp garlic powder

- ¼ tsp baking soda

- Salt

Stuffing

- ¼ onion, chopped

- 2 cloves of garlic, minced

- ¼ tomatoes, chopped

- ¼ small broccoli

- Salt

- Pepper

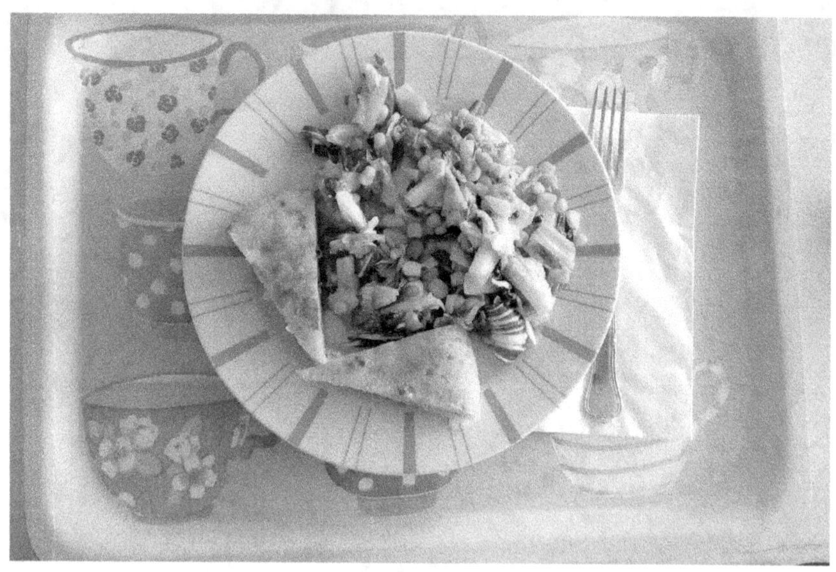

Methods:

1. Mix together all ingredients and add a pinch of salt to taste until a medium consistency or pancake-like consistency. Set aside for the baking soda to take effect.

2. Heat a non-stick pan or skillet with olive oil.

3. Saute the onion and garlic until they are soft and slightly brown in colour then add in the broccoli as well as salt and pepper to taste. Set aside for a while in a plate.

4. Reuse the same pan or skillet by adding a bit of oil and pour the omelette batter into it.

5. Add the sautéed onion, garlic and broccoli, as well as chopped tomatoes onto the batter. Leave it until there are bubbles around the edges before folding the omelette.

6. After folding the omelette, turn off the stove and cover it with a lid to allow it to steam up.

7. Serve it as it is or add some garnish on top of it.

<u>Health fact</u>

- ✓ Chickpea is a good substitute for meat as it is rich in protein. Not only that, it is also good to improve digestion and lower the risk of many diseases.

- ✓ White eggs can be substituted with chickpea liquid. Chickpea liquid comes from the liquid used to cook chickpea, added with some lemon juice. It works the same way as egg whites and could even be used in baking to produce meringue.

BREAKFAST SCRAMBLE

Ingredients:

- 1 tbsp coconut oil

- ¼ cup diced white onion

- 2 cloves of garlic, minced

- 1 cup of tofu

- Half lemon juices

- Salt and pepper

Methods:

1. Crumble tofu with a fork in a small bowl then add in lemon juice and salt and pepper for seasoning.

2. Heat and coconut oil into a skillet or a non-stick pan, then saute the onion and minced garlic until fragrant, soft and golden brown.

3. Mix the tofu mixture with the sautéed onion and garlic for 2-3 minutes until the tofu is warm enough thoroughly.

4. Serve as it is or with bread for your breakfast.

Health fact

✓ Tofu is great for breast cancer survivors as it prevents the recurrence of breast cancer. However, this fact is not firm enough to be suggested to breast cancer survivors.

✓ Soy is also associated to kidney function, particularly those with kidney failures. In general, proteins contained in soy could improve the renal function.

PEANUT BUTTER WITH RASPBERRY JAM PORRIDGE

Ingredients:

- ½ cup mixture of nuts, seeds and coconuts

- 2/3 cups rolled oats

- 2 tbsp unsweetened peanut butter

- 1 ½ cup plant-based milk (soy milk, almond milk, etc.)

- ¼ cup raspberries

- 2 tbsp maple syrup

- ¼ cup mixture of berries (strawberries, blueberries, raspberries, etc.) - optional

Methods:

1. For the jam, mash the raspberries with a fork or a spoon and add in maple syrup for sweetness. Set aside for a while in a small bowl.

2. Mix together the mixture of nuts, seeds and coconuts, rolled oats, peanut butter and milk in a pan and boil for two minutes to reduce it to simmer. Constantly stir the porridge while cooking to ensure that it doesn't stick to the pan.

3. Top the porridge with the jam and serve with fresh berries or just as it is.

Health fact

✓ Peanut butter is good for improving heart health, aid in weight-loss and bodybuilding as it contains protein which is crucial to build and repair the muscles. For young women, peanut butter is a good source to lower benign breast cancer (BBD) risks which could stimulate the risk of breast cancer.

✓ When choosing jams for plant-based diet, choose the one without added sugar as the main point of this diet is not to consume any type of sugars at all. Instead, the main objective is to use only plant-based ingredients in our food. A good substitute of sugars for this diet is maple syrup.

TOAST WITH AVOCADO AND SCRAMBLED TOFU

Ingredients:

- ½ avocado, sliced

- ½ tsp turmeric powder

- 2 tbsp olive oil

- 1 slice wholemeal bread, toasted

- 3 blocks of tofu

- 2 cloves of garlic, finely chopped

- 1 medium-sized tomato, diced

- 1 whole spring onion, chopped

- 2 chilli, finely chopped

- Salt and pepper

Methods:

1. Crumble the tofu with a fork until it resembles a scrambled egg. Set aside.

2. Put olive oil into a skillet or a pan and let it heat up for 30 seconds over medium heat, then put in the garlic, spring onion and chilli into the pan and Saute until fragrant.

3. Next add in crumbled tofu, turmeric powder, salt and pepper. Mix together with the other ingredients until tofu is cooked

and well combined. Turn off the heat and leave to cool for 5-10 minutes.

4. Finally, line up sliced avocado on top of the toasted bread then top it with the crumbled tofu.

5. Sprinkle with chilli flakes and it is ready to serve.

Health fact

✓ Avocados are rich in nutrients as they contain magnesium, potassium, vitamin C, vitamin E, vitamin K and vitamin B-6. Vitamin K in avocados are good to prevent osteoporosis. Other health benefits of avocados are reducing the risk of depression, cancer, heart disease and other chronic diseases.

✓ Ground pepper is a good seasoning agent filled with plenty of health benefits such as relieving cold and cures migraine. It is commonly added in soups and is best consumed during winter or cold weather.

FRENCH TOAST WITH BANANA CREAM AND BLUEBERRY

Ingredients:

Toast

- 1 slice of whole meal bread

- ¼ cup plant-based milk (soy milk, almond milk, etc.)

- ½ tbsp plain floor

- ½ tbsp maple syrup

- ½ tbsp vanilla extract

Topping

- 1 medium-sized banana

- ½ cup blueberries

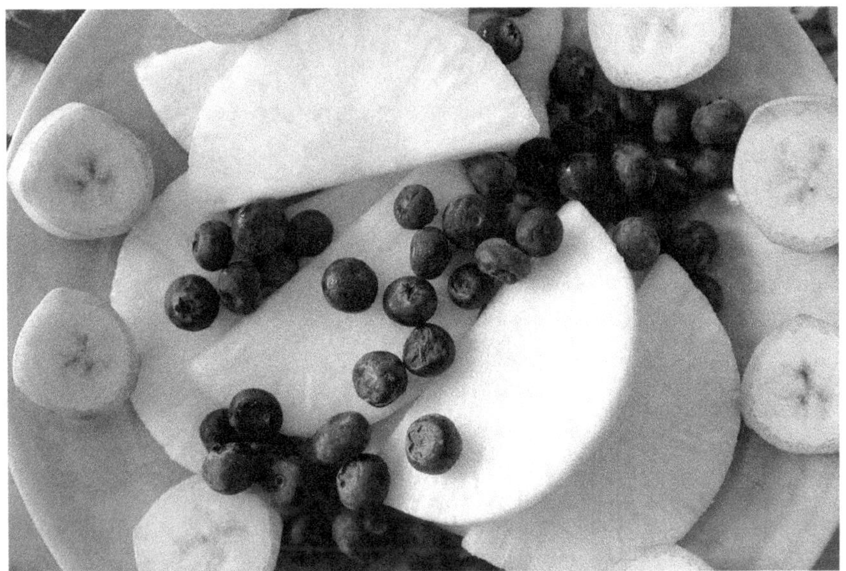

Methods:

1. For the toast, mix all ingredients together until well-combined then dip in the bread into the mixture so that it soaks up all of it.

2. Heat a non-stick pan with olive oil for 30 seconds then fry the soaked toast until both sides are crispy and golden brown then turn off the heat.

3. For the topping, blend the banana until smooth.

4. Serve the toast on a plate and top it with the smoothed banana and some blueberries.

<u>Health fact</u>

✓ Plain flour contains less fibre than wheat flour.

✓ Maple syrup contains zinc and manganese which are great for your immunity and as a source of energy respectively. Maple syrup is produced from a sugar maple tree which is tapped then boiled until slightly thicken. Maple syrup has a slightly runnier consistency than honey.

ROASTED GARLIC POTATOES

Ingredients:

- 4 medium-sized potatoes

- ¼ tbsp olive oil

- ½ tsp salt

- 1 tsp ground black pepper

- 2 tbsp minced garlic

- 2 tbsp minced parsley

Methods:

1. Prepare a baking tin and preheat the oven to 200-210 degree Celsius.

2. Cut the potatoes into cubes and then put them into a bowl with salt, olive oil, black pepper, and garlic. Toss all ingredients until they are well combined.

3. Spread the well-mixed potatoes and herbs on a baking tin evenly and put them into the oven to be roasted for about 45 minutes until 1 hour, or until golden brown. Flip every 15 minutes in order to get an even cooking.

4. Garnish the potatoes with parsley and it is ready to be served in a salad bowl.

Health fact

- ✓ Potatoes contain more potassium than that in bananas, which are good to strengthen our bone, muscle and improve cardiovascular health. It also contains about the same amount of vitamin C needed by our body per day.

- ✓ Baking your food is much healthier than frying because less oil is used in baking. While for frying, about twice as much oil is needed to stir fry your dishes which could lead to an excessive fat intake.

FRUITY BANANA SPLIT

Ingredients:

- 1 banana, cut in half

- 1 tbsp Greek yogurt

- ¼ cup raspberries

- ¼ cup blackberries

- Granola or any other nuts

- Dark chocolate chips

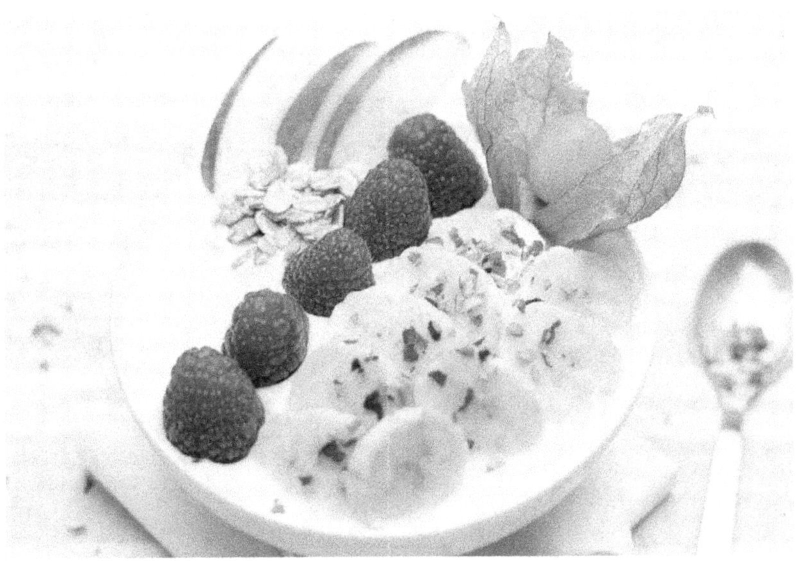

Methods:

1. Place the halved banana into a long dessert bowl or plate.

2. Spread some Greek yogurt on top of the banana, no need to be spread evenly right on top.

3. Add the 3-4 berries each on top of the yogurt then sprinkle some granola or nuts with dark chocolate chips on top.

4. Ready to be served as your fruit breakfast.

<u>Health fact</u>

✓ Greek yogurt is a good source of calcium which helps in bone development and contains probiotics which helps in healthy bacterial balance inside the bowel system.

✓ Nuts are a good alternative to meat or other animal-based proteins but should be taken in a moderate amount as they are high in calories.

✓ Walnuts are a good source of fat for those who are underweight and that it contains Omega 3 which is commonly found in fish.

SIMPLE PEANUT BUTTER BREAKFAST BAR

Ingredients:

- 1 ½ cup pitted dates

- ½ cup unsweetened creamy peanut butter

- ½ cup rolled oats

- 2 tbsp maple syrup (for sweetness)

Methods:

1. Soak the dates in warm water to soften them up and then drain the water.
2. In a blender, put in the dates, peanut butter and maple syrup until smooth.
3. Add in rolled oats into the mixture and fold over until well combined. If you prefer a more solid bar, add more oats into the mixture.
4. Spread the peanut butter mixtures evenly onto a baking tin of any sizes, depending on your preferred thickness and then put it into the freezer to set for 6-7 hours.
5. After 6-7 hours, slice the bars into 8-10 pieces and keep in an airtight container for easy keeping in the freezer. The bars should last up to 6 months.

<u>Health fact</u>

- ✓ Dates are a good source of energy and could keep you full throughout the day and prevents overeating.

✓ Diabetic patients are encouraged to consume dates as they are great to balance the sugar in their blood, as well as having a low GI value. The consumption of dates is also good before and after fasting to regulate the blood sugar level.

SALAD AND SOUP RECIPES

Salad and soups are the two food that great to be consumed at any time of the day, and that the method of preparation of respective foods are also very simple and less time consuming compared to other foods. This section provides you with a variety of salad and soup recipes suitable to be consumed as suggested in the diet plan. In the diet plan, salads and soups are suggested as meals for lunch, dinner and snack. The following list will include various interesting recipes for salads and soups according to the food plan.

Salads

1. Spinach with strawberry salad
2. Greek pasta salad
3. Winter vegetables salad
4. Blood orange salad
5. Farro lentil salad
6. Potato salad
7. Carrot and shredded beet salad
8. Classic coleslaw
9. Corn salad
10. Plant sausages with rice salad
11. Carrot salad
12. Crunchy silverbeet slaw

Soups

1. Tomato with tofu soup
2. Miso soup
3. Mushroom and broccoli soup

4. <u>Leek potato soup</u>
5. <u>Chickpea noodle soup</u>
6. <u>Carrot soup with fresh ginger</u>
7. <u>Shiitake mushroom with beansprouts and chilli soup</u>
8. <u>Creamy pumpkin soup</u>
9. <u>Butternut squash soup with spices</u>
10. <u>Spinach soup with mint</u>
11. <u>Spicy black beans with corn soup</u>

SPINACH WITH STRAWBERRY SALAD

Ingredients:

- 4 cups spinach (about 2 bunches – washed with water, rinsed and torn apart)

- 4 cups strawberry (sliced)

- ½ cup extra virgin olive oil

- ¼ tsp paprika

- 2 tbsp sesame seeds

- Toasted almonds or any nuts (optional)

- Salt and pepper

Methods:

1. Toss together the spinach and sliced strawberry in a salad bowl.

2. On a separate, small dish, mix together the ingredients for the salad dressing - olive oil, paprika and sesame seeds.

3. Pour the salad dressing into the salad bowl and toss the salad again until well incorporated with the dressing. Sprinkle some almonds or any nuts if you prefer some crunchiness in your salad and season with salt and pepper.

4. Serve to be eaten with a French toasted bread or as it is.

Health fact

- ✓ Spinach are a good source of vitamin A and C which fights against chronic diseases such as cancers- specifically colon and breast cancer.

- ✓ Spinach also could produce collagen which are great for the skin which could reduce skin aging.

- ✓ Doctors recommends consuming one cup of spinach a day as they could regulate your blood sugar level and prevent constipation or other digestive problems.

GREEK PASTA SALAD

Ingredients:

- 4 cups of dry plant-based pasta – preferably penne or rotini pasta, boiled

- 1 ½ cup cucumber, diced

- 1 green bell pepper, diced

- ½ cup cherry tomatoes

- ½ cup parsley, finely chopped

- ¼ tbsp extra virgin olive oil

- ½ orange, squeezed for the juice

- ¼ tsp paprika

- Salt and pepper

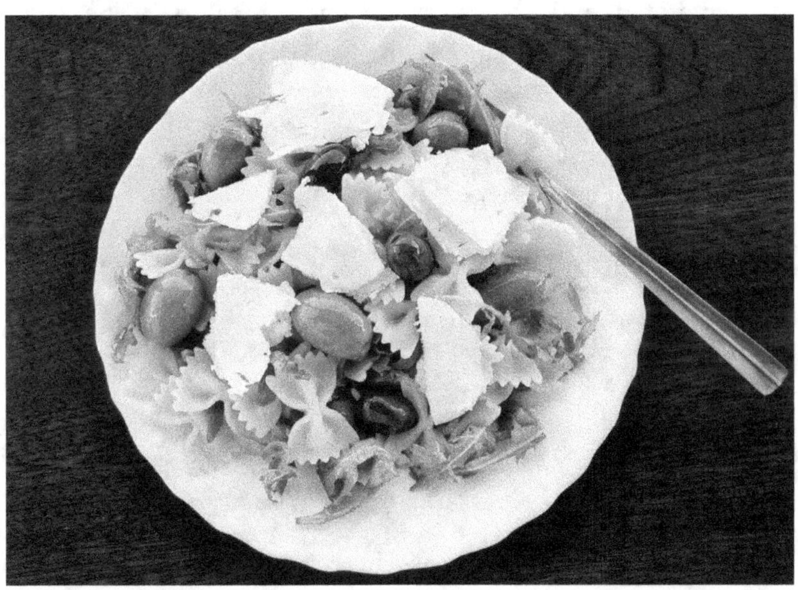

Methods:

1. In a salad bowl, toss together the pasta, cucumber, bell pepper and cherry tomatoes until well combined.

2. For the dressing, mix together the olive oil, orange juice, paprika and salt and pepper. Pour the mixture over the pasta and vegetables until well incorporated.

3. Garnish with some parsley and serve.

Health fact

✓ Plant-based pasta is commonly found in the organic section of the supermarkets and is used to be not so popular back then. However, thanks to the growing concern of eating healthy food, plant-based pasta can now be found along with the regular pasta.

✓ Cucumber contains about 96% of water. It could keep you hydrated and is also very low in calorie. The calorie content of a cucumber is about 15-16 calories.

WINTER VEGETABLES SALAD

Ingredients:

- 1 cup frozen chickpeas

- 1 medium-sized green apple, sliced

- 15 small lettuce leaves

- ¼ cup broccoli florets

- ¼ cup baby carrots

- ¼ cup cauliflower florets

- 2 tbsp extra virgin olive oil

- 1 small garlic clove, minced or grated finely

- Salt and pepper

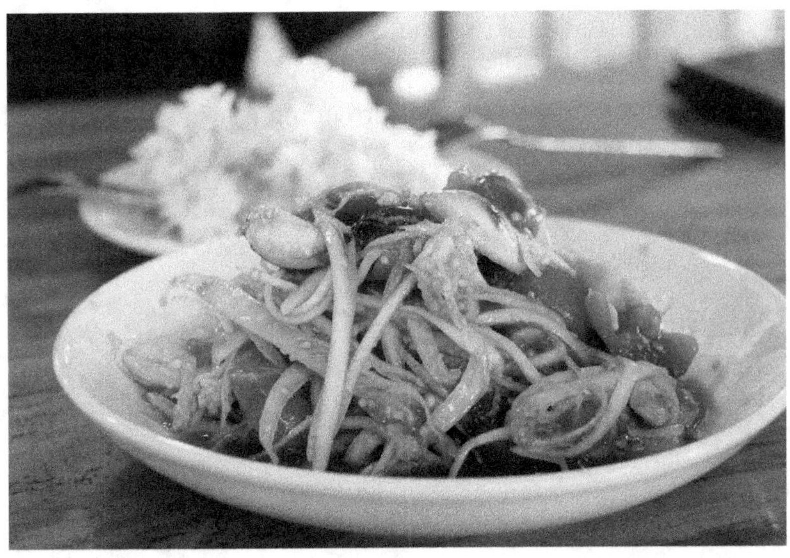

Methods:

1. Defrost the chickpeas for 2-3 minutes.

2. In a large salad bowl, add chickpeas, apple, lettuce, broccoli, carrots, and cauliflower and then toss them together until well combined.

3. For the dressing, mix together olive oil, garlic and some salt and pepper and then pour over the salad. Toss the salad again until well-incorporated. Could be served and eaten immediately or keep in the fridge for a few minutes if you prefer to eat it cool.

<u>Health fact</u>

✓ Salad are a better option to be consumed as a light snack in place of other sweet and salty snacks such as chips and chocolate as they are full of nutrients and low in calorie.

✓ Extra virgin olive oils are great for salad dressing because they are flavoured specially to be used for salad dressing, uncooked sauces or for drizzles. They come with many healthy goodness such as providing a healthy saturated fat in your diet.

BLOOD ORANGE SALAD

Ingredients:

- 3-4 blood oranges

- ¼ small-sized red onion, thinly sliced

- 2 tbsp extra virgin olive oil

- Fresh mint (optional)

- Salt and pepper

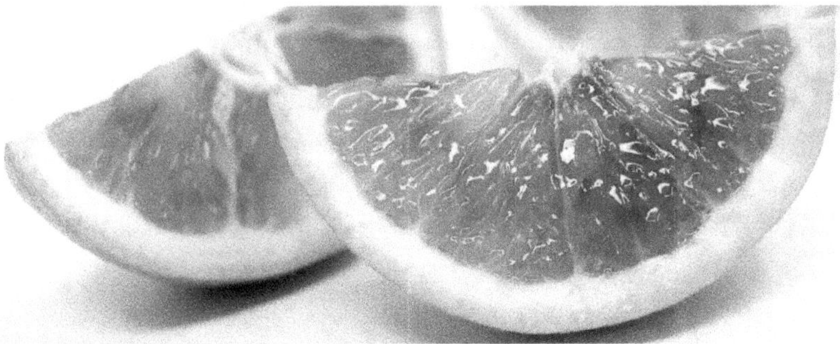

Methods:

1. Chill the oranges in the fridge for 1-2 hours, then peel and slice roughly for about ½ inches.

2. In a salad bowl, toss the oranges and red onion together until well incorporated, then add salt and pepper to taste. Top with some fresh mint for garnish and your salad is ready to be indulged.

<u>Health fact</u>

✓ Blood orange contains a substance called anthocyanins which acts as an antioxidant, and thus good to be consumed often for a better and young-looking skin. Not only that, this substance could also help in preventing cancers, infections from bacteria, diabetes and heart diseases.

✓ Despite being in the fruit class, blood orange is also a good source of calcium which is beneficial for bones and teeth, particularly in term of strength. Therefore, blood orange is good replacement for dairy products especially milk.

✓ There are differences in the antioxidants level between a blood orange and a regular orange. Blood orange contains a much higher antioxidants level compared to the regular one, which is why it is preferable to use this orange in our diet.

FARRO LENTIL SALAD

Ingredients:

- 3 cups of cooked farro

- 1 cup of cooked lentils

- 1 clove of minced garlic

- 2 tbsp lemon juice

- ½ cup cherry tomatoes, halved

- ¼ cup yellow bell pepper

- ¼ cup red bell pepper

- ¼ cup extra virgin olive oil

- Salt and pepper

Methods:

1. In a salad bowl, toss together the farro, lentils, tomatoes and the bell peppers until well combined.

2. For the dressing, whisk together minced garlic, lemon juice, olive oil, salt and pepper in a small dish then pour on top of combined salad. Toss the salad again until well combined with the dressing.

3. Serve with wholemeal bread or eat as it is.

Health fact

- ✓ Farro is an excellent source to keep your colon healthy as it contains a high level of fibre and protein. This indicates that farro is as good as rice or other grains, but only healthier and much better. It is a good alternative to both grains as they are greatly beneficial for keeping your body stay in shape.

- ✓ Generally, garlic is very low in calorie but could provide a highly nutritious benefits to our health such as lowering the cholesterol level, which in turn could reduce the risk of getting a heart disease.

- ✓ There are about 25% of protein in lentils that makes it a good replacement to meat.

POTATO SALAD

Ingredients:

- 5 medium-sized potatoes

- 1 medium-sized red onion, thinly sliced

- 1 bell peppers, sliced (any one colour; red or yellow or green)

- ½ cup celery, roughly chopped

- 1 tsp lemon juice

- 1 tbsp mustard

- 1 tbsp extra virgin olive oil

- 3 cloves garlic, minced

- Cashews (roasted or raw)

- Salt and pepper

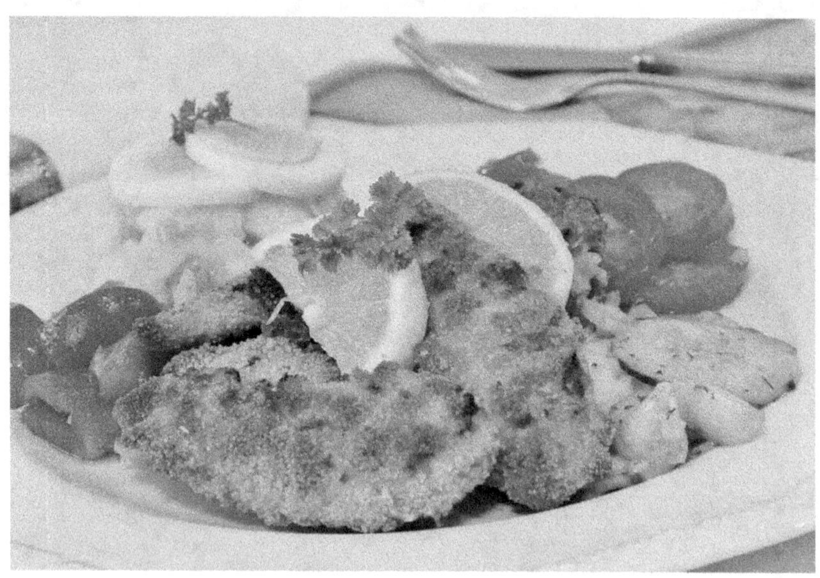

Methods:

1. Boil the potatoes, with or without skin (depending on your preference), for 15-20 minutes or until they can be cut through using a knife or a spoon. Drain and set aside to let cool.

2. While waiting for the potatoes to be cooled, you could prepare the dressing by adding in the mustard, olive oil, lemon juice, garlic and salt and pepper by whisking all of these ingredients together in a small dish or bowl. Set aside.

3. Cut the potatoes into bite-sized pieces then put them in a large salad bowl. Add in the red onion, peppers and celery and toss them together until well incorporated. Pour the salad dressing and then toss again, then top with some cashews to add a crunchy taste to your salad.

Health fact

- ✓ Celery could reduce and prevent inflammation in the body such as arthritis and osteoporosis.

- ✓ Celery is rich in vitamins A, C and K which are low in its GI value and sodium content, thus could regulate your blood sugar level.

CARROT AND SHREDDED BEET SALAD

Ingredients:

- 2 raw beets, peeled and grated

- 2 medium-sized carrots, peeled and grated

- ½ tbsp maple syrup

- 1 tbsp extra virgin olive oil

- ¼ cup lemon juice

- ¼ tsp cinnamon, grounded

- ½ tsp coriander, grounded

- ¼ tsp paprika

- Parsley (optional)

- Salt and pepper

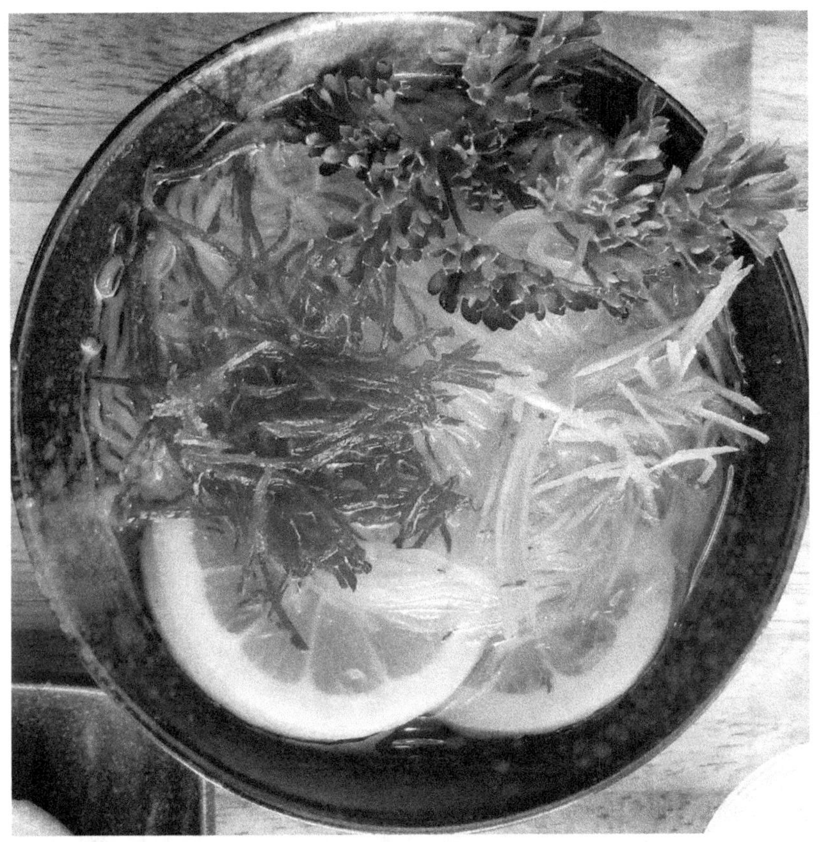

Methods:

1. In a medium-sized bowl, toss together the beets and carrots until well combined.

2. For the dressing, whisk together the maple syrup, olive oil, lemon juice, cinnamon, coriander, paprika and salt and pepper until well mixed then pour over the vegetables and toss again until well incorporated. Garnish with some finely chopped parsley before serving.

Health fact

- ✓ Beets are a good source of vitamin C which is well-known for its function in immunity and provide healthy skin. Other than that, beets are also linked to factors that contributed to an improved performance during exercises, blood flow as well as reducing the blood pressure.

- ✓ Carrots has long been associated with improving the vision, specifically our night vision.

- ✓ Fruit juice contains more sugars than a whole fruit, thus making it to have more calorie content. This is due to the fact that fruit juice does not contain any fibre which is supposed to slow down the sugar absorption in our body.

CLASSIC COLESLAW

Ingredients:

- ½ purple cabbage, thinly sliced

- ½ small red onion, thinly sliced

- 2 cups shredded carrots

- 1 ½ cup cherry tomatoes, halved

- 2 cloves garlic, finely chopped

- 2 tbsp extra virgin olive oil

- ¼ tbsp mustard

- ¼ tbsp maple syrup

- ½ tbsp orange or lemon juice

- Salt and pepper

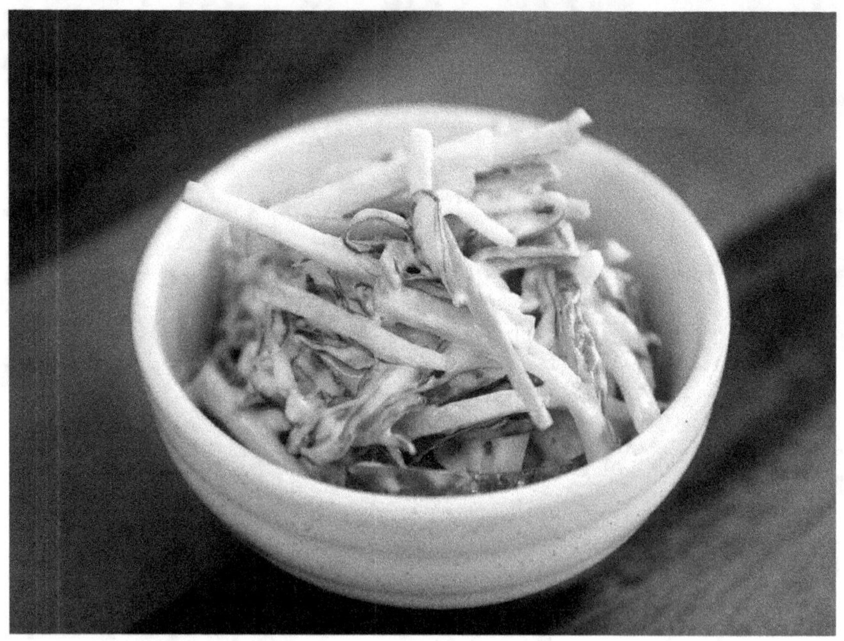

Methods:

1. In a medium bowl, add in the cabbage, red onion, carrots and tomatoes and toss until well combined then set aside to prepare for the dressing.

2. In a small bowl, add in the olive oil, mustard, maple syrup, orange or lemon juice, garlic, salt and pepper, and whisk together until well mixed. Combine the salad dressing with the vegetables and mix together until they are evenly covered with the dressing.

3. Serve or keep in the fridge for up to 3 days. Best eaten when cold.

Health fact

- ✓ The purple colour of the purple cabbage has a high concentration of a substance called anthocyanin polyphenols which makes it have more nutrients than the regular, green cabbage. This substance contains a high level of antioxidants which is great for the skin and eliminate waste substances in the body easier.

- ✓ There are only about 28 calories for 1 cup of chopped purple cabbage and that it contains about 90% of water. The high-water content in purple cabbage or other regular cabbages is one of the reasons why you could get the crunchiness while eating them raw.

CORN SALAD

Ingredients:

- 6 ears of corn, removed from its husk

- ½ small-sized red onion, sliced thinly

- 3 tbsp extra virgin olive oil

- ½ cup basil leaves, julienned

- Salt and pepper

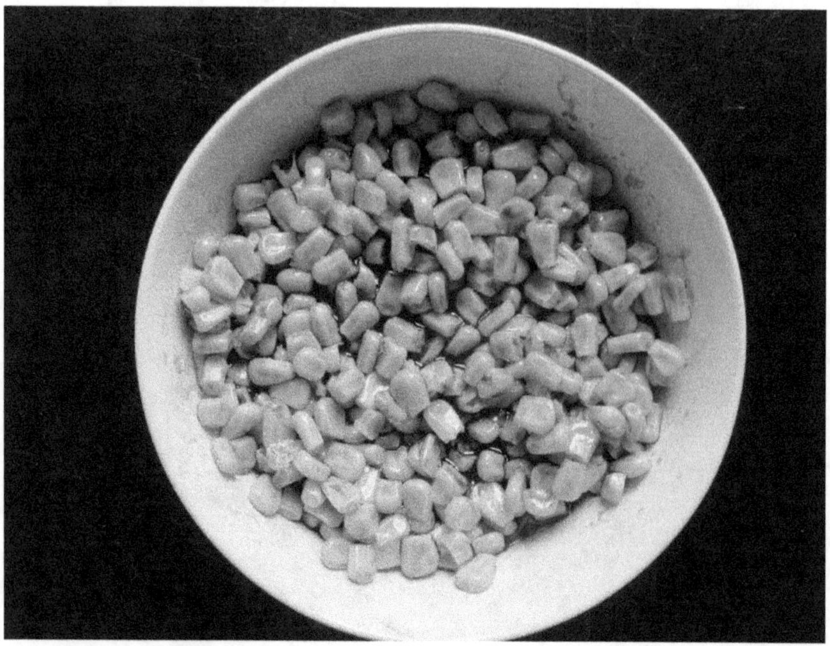

Methods:

1. In a large pot, put in the corn and some water enough to cover the corn. Then add a pinch of salt into the pot and let

it cook for 3 minutes. Next, drain the water and cool down the corn in a bowl with ice water to sustain its colour and stop the cooking process. In a flat surface, use your knife to scrap the corn off of its corncob then add the corn into a medium bowl. Then add red onion into the bowl and toss them together until well combined.

2. In a small bowl, mix together the olive oil and basil leaves, as well as some salt and pepper to taste. Then pour the dressing over the corn and red onion mixture in the other bowl. Toss all ingredients together until evenly combined.

Health fact

✓ An ear of corn contains only 96 calories. Not only that, it could help you to resist hunger for almost throughout the day. Moreover, the lutein and zeaxanthin content commonly found in corns could sustain your eye vision.

✓ Salads which are made up of fresh ingredients are healthier than those made with days old ingredients because the nutritional contents are still intact in fresh ingredients, and you could still get the crunchiness in every bite. The latter ingredients, however, may have lost some of their nutritional value due to it being kept for so long. Nevertheless, you could use either one depending on their availability in your storage, but a much better one is the ones that are fresh.

PLANT SAUSAGES WITH RICE SALAD

Ingredients:

Plant-based sausages

- 3 cups of chickpeas, cooked

- 2 cups wheat flour

- 4 cloves garlic, thinly sliced

- 1 tbsp tomato paste

- ½ large red onion, thinly sliced

- ½ tbsp cumin

- ½ tbsp thyme

- ½ tbsp paprika

- Salt and pepper

- Corn oil (for Saute)

Salad

- 2 cups of cooked rice (white or brown rice)

- ½ cucumber, diced

- ½ cup corn, cooked

- ½ cup cherry tomatoes, halved

- ½ tbsp extra virgin olive oil

- ½ tsp smoked paprika

- ½ tbsp coriander

- Salt and pepper

Methods:

For the sausages:

1. Heat the corn oil in a skillet and then add in the garlic, red onion and cumin and Saute until fragrant and soften. Turn off the heat and set aside.

2. In a food processor, put in the chickpeas, tomato paste, sautéed mixtures, tomato paste, thyme, paprika, salt and pepper, blend until smooth. Then add in wheat flour into the mixture until well combined and less sticky.

3. On a flat surface, roll over the sausage dough and shape it like an actual sausage. Grill with some oil and set aside to make the salad.

For the salad:

1. In a large bowl, mix together the rice, cucumber, corn and cherry tomatoes until well combined. Set aside to make the dressing.

2. For the dressing, mix together the olive oil, paprika, coriander and salt and pepper in a small bowl then pour over the rice and vegetables in the other bowl. Toss the salad together until well combined.

3. Serve the salad with the plant-based sausages and you're ready to eat. Best eaten for lunch or dinner.

Health fact

- ✓ The typical meat sausages are commonly made using processed meat, including unhealthy fat which could trigger heart diseases.

- ✓ Plant-based sausages are a better option for individuals who would like to reduce their red meat consumption or having meat withdrawal syndrome.

CARROT SALAD

Ingredients:

- 5 carrots, grated

- 2 shallots, sliced thinly

- 1 tbsp lemon juice

- 2 tbsp parsley, chopped

- 1 ½ tbsp extra virgin olive oil

- ½ tbsp plant-based syrup (e.g. maple syrup)

- Salt and pepper

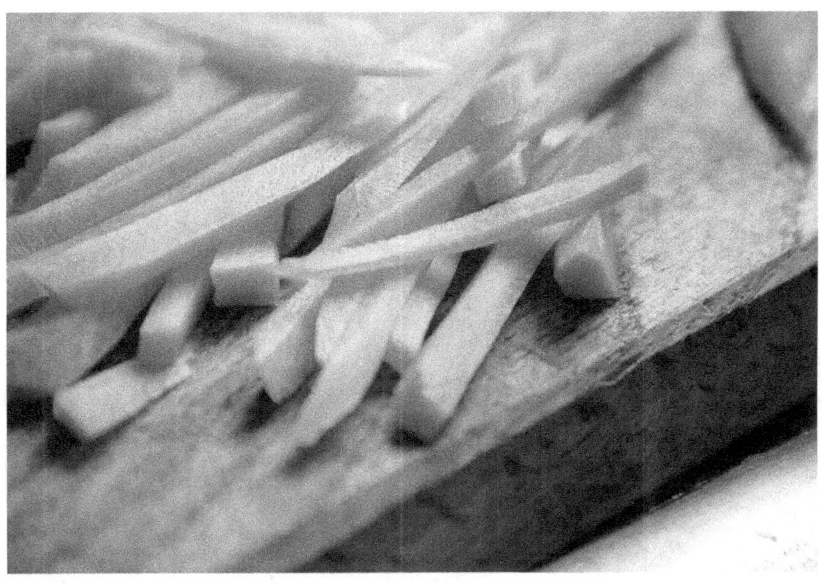

Methods:

1. In a large bowl, toss the carrots and shallots together until evenly mixed.

2. Add in the liquid ingredients such as lemon juice, olive oil and syrup. Then add some salt and pepper as well as chopped parsley then toss again until well incorporated.

3. Serve or keep in the fridge for up to 3 days.

Health fact

✓ Shallots are a good source of vitamin B6 which assist in the functionalities of the nervous and immune systems.

✓ The selenium content in shallots is good for protecting cells against aging and also could promote a healthy hair and skin.

✓ The store-bought salad dressings are not that healthy as they contain extra amount of salt and some sugar than the one you make at home. Salt do not have any calories, but it could retain water by absorbing the water and eventually make you gain some weight. This is why physicians highly recommend reducing the amount of daily sodium intake. The latest recommended sodium intake is 1600 mg.

CRUNCHY SILVERBEET SLAW

Ingredients:

- 1 bunch silverbeet, thinly sliced its leaves and stems

- 1 beetroot, peeled and julienned

- 1 green apple, peeled and julienned

- 2 celeries, thinly sliced

- ¼ cups roasted or raw walnuts

- 1 tsp chia seed

- ¼ cup extra virgin olive oil

- Salt and pepper

Methods:

1. Toss together the silverbeet, beetroot, apple and celeries until evenly mixed.

2. Drizzle some olive oil and sprinkle some chia seed into the salad. Add salt and pepper to taste. Then toss again until well combined.

3. Top with some roasted or raw walnuts and it is ready to eat. The salad could last up to 5 days if it is kept in the fridge.

<u>**Health fact**</u>

✓ Silverbeet can be eaten both raw and cooked. It is typically good for blood circulation and blood clotting. Other than that, the manganese content in silverbeet could also assist in regulating the functionalities of the nerves and brain.

✓ Green apples are much better than the red ones for weight loss because it has less carbohydrates and sugars than the latter. However, these differences are too small in comparison and either one apple could work for your weight-loss diet.

TOMATO WITH TOFU SOUP

Ingredients:

- 3 tomatoes, cut into quarters

- 1 ½ tofu blocks, cubed

- 1 cloves garlic, thinly sliced

- 2 shallots, thinly sliced

- 1 tbsp finely chopped coriander

- 1 ½ tbsp olive oil

- 1 cup plain water

- Salt and pepper

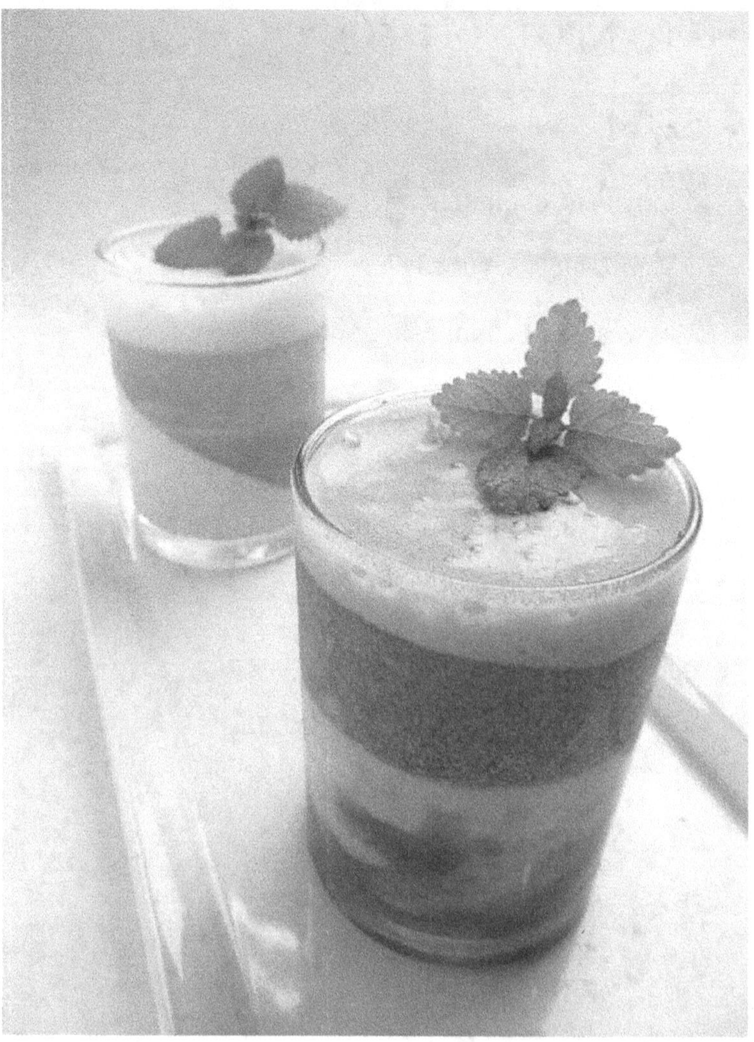

Methods:

1. In a medium pot, heat the olive oil and Saute the garlic and shallots until fragrant and slightly brownish.

2. Add in the plain water and leave to boil over a medium heat. To make it boil faster, cover the pot. When the water boils, lower the heat and add in the tomatoes and tofu. Add some

salt and pepper to taste and leave to boil again for about 5 minutes.

3. Serve in a large bowl and garnish with come coriander. Best eaten as a snack or comfort food.

Health fact

- ✓ Extra virgin olive oil is the healthiest type of olive oil. However, for cooking and grilling, an extra light olive oil is the most suitable one because it could last higher in high temperatures due to its high smoke point. Extra virgin olive oil however could burn easily in high temperatures, making it less suitable for cooking and grilling.

- ✓ Watery foods like soups or chowders typically contains high amount of salt. This is because since it has to be added with water, cooks need to ensure that their food does not taste plain, so salt is added to be diffused with water. If you are attempting to live healthy, try to reduce the amount of salt in your soups or in any other food and you will see a big difference upon yourself.

MISO SOUP

Ingredients:

Vegetable broth

- 2 carrots, grated

- 2 celery sticks, chopped

- 1 whole red onion, thinly sliced with skin

- 1 whole garlic, roughly chopped with skin

- 1 bay leaf

- 1 sheet dried seaweed

- ½ tbsp thyme

- ½ tbsp parsley

- ½ tbsp rosemary

- 10 cups water

- Olive oil

- Salt and pepper

Miso soup

- ½ cup green onion, chopped

- ½ cup firm tofu

- 4 tbsp fermented soybean paste (available at Asian supermarkets)

- 3 cups hot water

- 3 cups vegetable broth

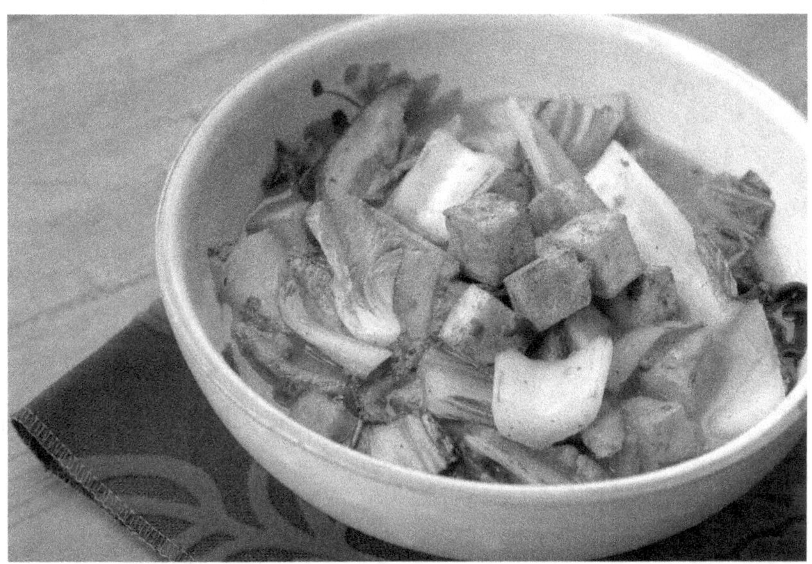

Methods:

For the broth:

1. Heat olive oil in a large pot, add in carrots, celery, onion, garlic, thyme, parsley and rosemary and Saute until fragrant and soft and tender. Next, add a bay leaf, seaweed and water as well as some salt and pepper. Leave to simmer for 1-2 hours or longer, over a medium heat. Cover with a lid.

2. After 1-2 hours, turn off the heat then strain the vegetables and store the broth in a large glass jar for later use. Store in a fridge to last up to 2 months.

For the miso:

1. Take some vegetable broth and fill in a medium pot and turn on the heat at a medium level.

2. In a small bowl, whisk the fermented bean paste (or also known as miso paste) with hot water to avoid the mixture from being clumpy, then add into the vegetable broth.

3. Add in the green onion and firm tofu and leave to simmer for 15-20 minutes before being served in a medium bowl. Best eaten as a side dish for lunch or dinner.

<u>Health fact</u>

✓ Miso provides us with good bacteria which is great for our gut health. This is due to its nature of being a fermented food. Furthermore, a healthy gut could also improve our mental and physical health in return.

✓ Japanese foods are commonly healthy and low calorie. It is actually very uncommon to see a fat Japanese. This is because the Japanese really emphasise on healthy diet and exercising is the key to live happily.

MUSHROOM AND BROCCOLI SOUP

Ingredients:

- 2 cups button mushroom, thinly sliced

- 2 cups broccoli florets

- 1 tbsp soy sauce

- 1 tbsp canola or olive oil

- 2 celery sticks, finely chopped

- ½ medium-sized red onion, finely chopped

- 1 garlic clove, minced

- 1 cup vegetable broth

- 2 cups water

- 2 tbsp lemon juice

- Salt and pepper

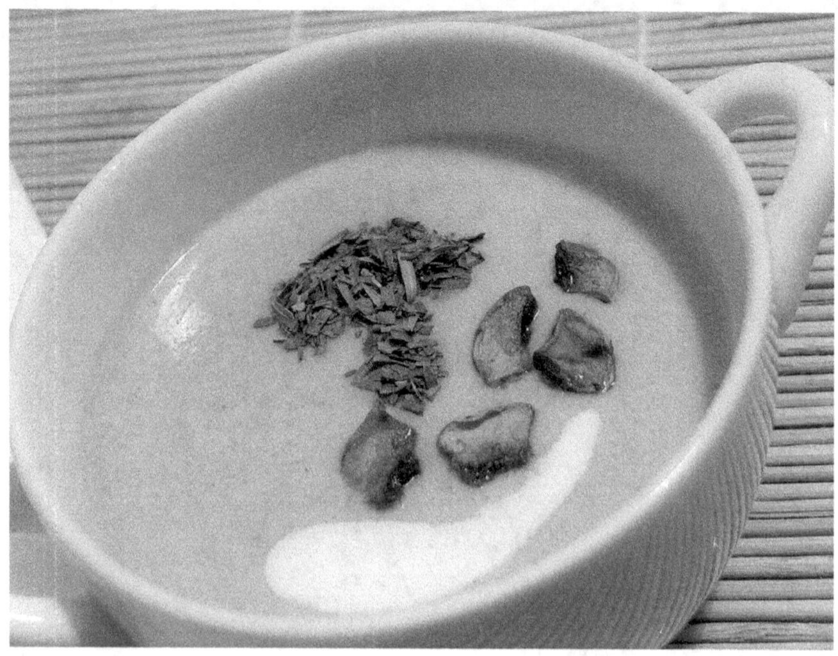

Methods:

1. Heat oil in a medium pot and Saute the mushroom until softened for 5 minutes then add in the soy sauce. Remove from the pot and set aside.

2. Next, in the same pot, put in the celery, onion, garlic, vegetable broth, and water. Then bring to a simmer over a medium heat for 30 minutes. Let cool for 10 minutes.

3. After 10 minutes of cooling, pour the vegetables mixture into a blender or food processor and puree until smooth then add it back into the pot. Add in the sautéed mushroom and broccoli florets and stir gently, bringing to a boil for 10 minutes. Lastly, add in some lemon juice as well as some salt and pepper to taste. Serve with wholemeal French bread or as it is and enjoy your snack.

Health fact

- ✓ Mushrooms are low in calorie and is good for diabetic patients and obese individuals as they have certain properties that could reduce the cholesterol level in the body. Lower cholesterol level means a healthier blood circulation and pressure.

- ✓ Deep fry foods are high in calorie and could increase the cholesterol level in our body. Increasing cholesterol level in our body could only lead to heart diseases, especially blockage in the heart artery. Other than that, obesity and high blood pressure could also occur when fried foods are consumed uncontrollably.

LEEK POTATO SOUP

Ingredients:

- 6 medium-sized potatoes, peeled

- 2 medium-sized leeks, sliced

- 1 tbsp olive oil

- 4 cups vegetable broth

- 4 cups plain water

- 1 tbsp rosemary

- 2 bay leaves

- 1 tbsp lemon juice

- Croutons (optional)

- Salt and pepper

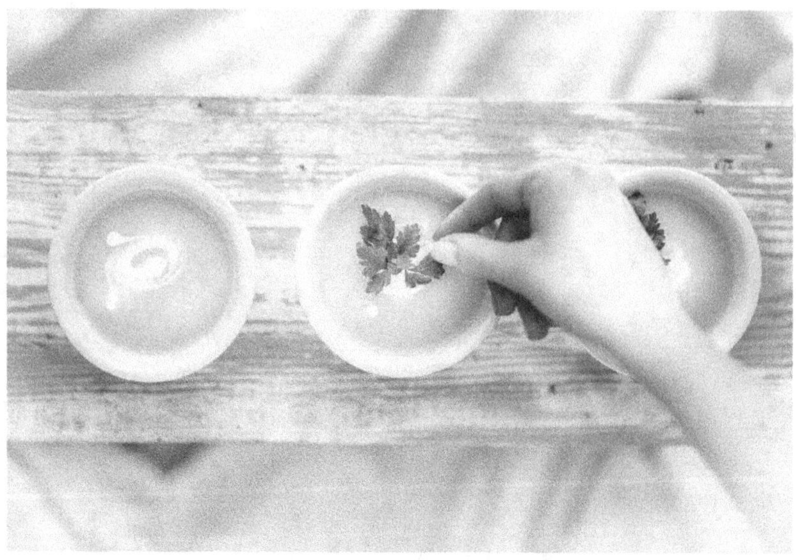

Methods:

1. In a large pot, heat olive oil then adds in the leeks to sautéed for 5 minutes or until softened. Put in the potatoes, broth, water, rosemary and bay leaves and leave to simmer over a low heat for 30 minutes until the potatoes are soft and tender for easy mashing.

2. Add some lemon juice and salt and pepper to taste then stir well. Leave to cool for about 10 minutes.

3. After cooling, add in the mixture into a blender and blend until smooth and creamy. Serve with some French bread or sprinkle some croutons on top for a crunchy taste. Enjoy your meal!

<u>Health fact</u>

- ✓ Leeks contain an excellent health benefits that the daily recommended intake is at least ½ cup per day. Leeks provide similar health benefits to onions and garlics such as preventing cancer and reducing inflammation.

- ✓ Croutons are typically baked and season with some salt and pepper. Seasoned croutons are found to have more nutrition than the unseasoned ones and it is better to choose the latter. For plant-based diet, you could use a whole wheat bread to make croutons.

CHICKPEA NOODLE SOUP

Ingredients:

- 1 clove garlic, minced

- ½ medium-sized red onion, chopped

- ½ carrot, peeled and thinly sliced

- 1 celery stick, thinly sliced

- 3 sprigs fresh thyme

- 1 bay leaf

- ¼ cup chickpea, cooked

- 1 ½ cup vegetable broth

- 1 cup rice noodles

- Salt and pepper

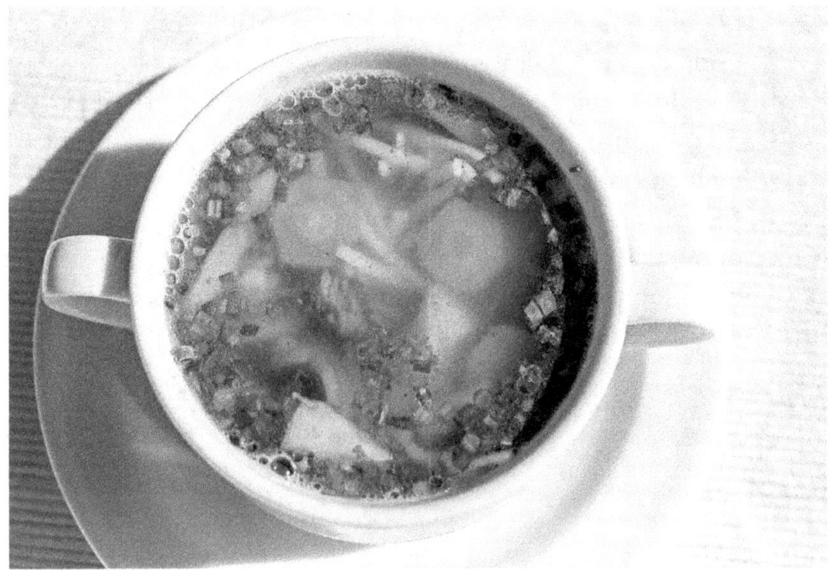

Methods:

1. Saute the garlic, onion, carrot, celery, thyme and bay leaf with heated olive oil in a pan or skillet until fragrant and softened. Add in the broth and bring to a boil over a medium heat.

2. Cook the noodles by soaking it in a hot water for about 10 minutes or until softened then rinsed with cold water for a chewy texture. Next add the noodles and the cooked chickpea into the vegetables and broth mixture and mix well.

3. Add in salt and pepper to taste before serving in a bowl.

<u>Health fact</u>

✓ Rice noodles are suitable for weight loss diet and as an alternative to pasta as they are solely made of rice flour and water, and without additional ingredients. The calories in rice noodles are also lower with 109 calories compared to egg noodles with 385 calories.

✓ The difference between calorific value and nutritional value is that calorific value measures the calorie content in foods, while nutritional value measures the amount of nutrition in foods. It is important to balance out both values so that you don't overconsumed any one of them. Both values are commonly included in the nutritional information label of your foods.

CARROT SOUP WITH FRESH GINGER

Ingredients:

- 3 carrots, chopped

- 1 garlic clove, thinly sliced

- 2 tbsp ginger, peeled and grated

- ½ medium-sized onion, thinly sliced

- ¼ cup coconut milk

- ¼ cup vegetable broth

- Olive oil

- Salt and pepper

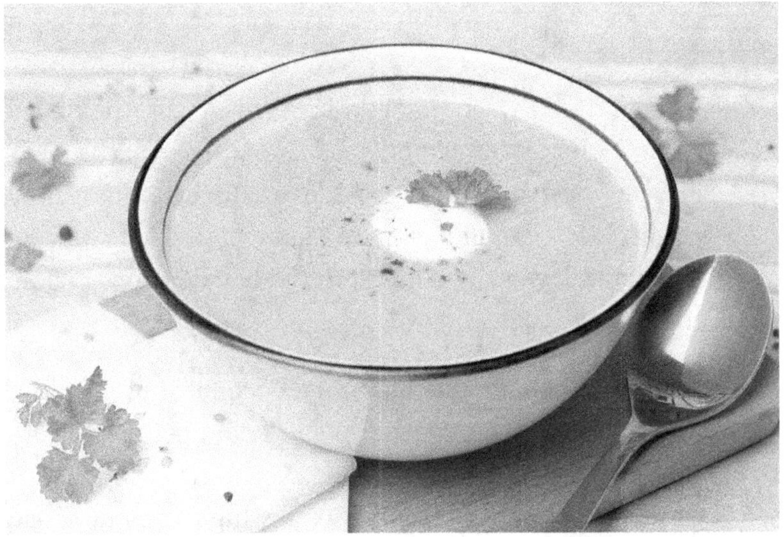

Methods:

1. Saute the onion and garlic with a heated oil in a medium pot until fragrant and softened.

2. Add in the carrots and ginger and stir until well incorporated for about 1 minutes, then add in the broth to bring to a boil.

3. Lower the heat then add in the coconut milk, simmer for about 15 minutes. Turn off the heat and allow to cool.

4. After cooling, put the mixture into a blender or food processor and blend until smooth and creamy. Then add some salt and pepper to taste. Drizzle some extra virgin olive oil on top.

5. Serve with bread or eat as it is. Best eaten for snack, lunch or dinner.

Health fact

✓ Coconut milk is commonly used in Asian cooking and should be taken in a moderate amount since it is high in calorie. However, it also provides health benefits mainly in weight loss, immune system and heart health. Coconut milk could lower the cholesterol level when consumed in a moderate amount.

✓ Apart from being made into milk, coconut water could also be drink raw. Fresh coconut water could help to lower the body temperature and in Asian countries, coconuts are typically used to cure fever. The high mineral content causes our body to rehydrate. In fact, drinking coconut water is the same as drinking isotonic water, only healthier without sugar.

SHIITAKE MUSHROOM WITH BEANSPROUTS AND CHILLI SOUP

Ingredients:

- 1 medium-sized onion, chopped
- 1 cup shiitake mushroom, washed
- 2 cloves garlic, thinly sliced
- ½ cup bean sprouts, washed
- ½ tbsp fresh chilli paste
- 3 cup plain water
- 2 tbsp olive oil
- Salt and pepper

Methods:

1. In a medium-sized pot, heat the olive oil and then add in the onion and garlic. Saute these two ingredients until fragrant and softened. Then add in the chilli paste and stir for about 2 minutes.

2. Add in plain water and bring to a boil.

3. Add in the mushroom and bean sprouts as well as some salt and pepper, lower the heat to bring it to a simmer for about 10-15 minutes.

4. Serve in a bowl. This soup is best eaten during winter as a snack, lunch or dinner menu.

<u>Health fact</u>

- ✓ Bean sprouts is fat-free and rich in vitamin C. The vitamin C content in bean sprouts could help to relief stress and anxiety, particularly in women who are more prone towards emotional deficiency. Not only that, the content of this vitamin as well as iron could boost the immune system too.

- ✓ According to a research, it is possible to use shiitake mushroom as a natural cancer treatment as it has several properties which could fight the cancer cells. Moreover, the damaged chromosomes caused by anticancer treatment could be treated by using lentinan which can be found in this mushroom.

CREAMY PUMPKIN SOUP

Ingredients:

- ¾ pumpkin, peeled and seeded

- ½ onion, chopped

- 1 garlic clove, chopped

- 2 cups vegetable broth

- ½ cup coconut milk

- Water (optional)

- Olive oil

- Salt and pepper

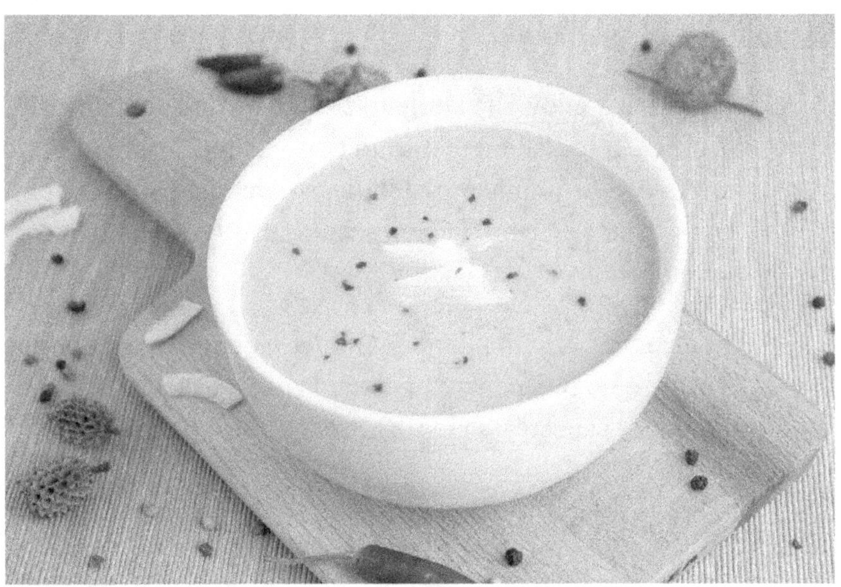

Methods:

1. Cut the pumpkin into bite-sized pieces.

2. Heat a pot with some olive oil over a medium heat, then add in the onion and garlic. Stir until golden brown or soft and tender.

3. Next add the broth, coconut milk, pumpkin and salt and pepper. Stir for 2 minutes then simmer for 20 minutes or until the pumpkin is soft and tender, over the same heat. If you think that it looks thick, add a little bit of water as per your preference. After simmering, set aside to cool.

4. Next, pour in the cooled soup mixture into a blender and blend until smooth. Serve in a bowl and eat with French bread or as it is.

<u>Health fact</u>

✓ Pumpkins are low in calorie (49 calories) and contains 94% of water. It is also a good source of vitamin A which could improve your immune system and fight against infections. Apart from that, this vitamin could also prevent sight loss as you get older.

✓ Carotenoids in pumpkins could act as antioxidants which in turn could reduce risk of certain cancers such as stomach and breast cancers.

BUTTERNUT SQUASH SOUP WITH SPICES

Ingredients:

- ¾ medium-sized butternut squash, peeled and seeded

- 3 shallots, thinly sliced

- 2 garlic cloves, thinly sliced

- 1 tsp maple syrup

- 2 cloves mint leaves (for garnish)

- 2 cups vegetable broth

- 2 cups plain water

- 3 tbsp olive oil (2 for Saute, 1 for drizzle)

- ¼ tsp ground nutmeg

- ¼ tsp ground cinnamon

- ¼ tsp paprika

- Salt and pepper

Methods:

1. Cut the butternut squash into bite-sized pieces.

2. In a large pot, heat olive oil over a medium-high heat then add in the shallots and garlic. Saute both ingredients until fragrant and slightly brown in colour.

3. Next, add in the broth and water as well as the butternut squash. Simmer for 20-25 minutes or until the butternut

squash is soft and tender, easy enough to be cut through using a spoon. Set aside to cool for about 10 minutes.

4. Then, pour the mixture into a blender then add in the nutmeg, cinnamon, paprika and salt and pepper before blending until smooth.

5. Serve in a bowl and drizzle some olive oil on top, as well as placing the mint leaves on top as a garnish.

Health fact

✓ Just like pumpkin, butternut squash also a good source of vitamin A which is good to reduce cancer. Other than that, it is also great for healthy skin and hair. However, butternut squash has a slightly higher calorie which is about 82 calories.

SPINACH SOUP WITH MINT

Ingredients:

- 10 stalks green spinach, removed from stalks and chopped

- 3 medium-sized potatoes, peeled and cubed

- ½ onion, chopped

- 3 garlic cloves, minced

- 2 cups vegetable broth

- ½ cup fresh mint, chopped

- Olive oil

- Salt and pepper

Methods:

1. Heat the olive oil in a large pot over a medium heat then add in the chopped onion. Saute until soft and tender, then add in the potatoes and garlic and stir for 5 minutes.

2. Next, add in the broth and bring to a boil. Cover the pot and bring to a simmer for 10 minutes or until the potatoes are soft and tender. Add in some the spinach and fresh mint, simmer again for about 2 minutes. Set aside to let it cool.

3. Pour the mixture into a blender then add some salt and pepper to taste. Blend until smooth and serve in a bowl.

Health fact

- ✓ Mints are commonly used to cure asthma, headache and memory loss. The minty aroma provides excellent relaxant and could relief the nose congestion. With that being said, mint could also improve the respiratory system which is why it is good to cure asthma. One of the reasons to use balm or minty oil to relief headache is because of its nature to produce a soothing feel towards the patients.

- ✓ Peeling to potato skin could lower its nutritional value. Potato skin contains more iron than its flesh. However, the nutrition contents both parts are equal.

SPICY BLACK BEANS WITH CORN SOUP

Ingredients:

- 1 cup dried black beans, rinsed

- ½ brown onion, chopped

- 2 cloves garlic, sliced thinly

- 1 celery stick, chopped

- 1 tsp cumin

- 1 tsp paprika

- ½ cup tomatoes, mashed

- 1 cup frozen corn, thawed

- 2 chillies, chopped

- 5 cups plain water

- Coriander (for garnish)

- Olive oil

- Salt and pepper

Methods:

1. In a medium pot, put in the black beans together with some water enough to cover the surface. Bring to a boil over a medium heat for about 5-10 minutes then drain. Set aside to prepare for other ingredients.

2. Heat a skillet or a non-stick pan with olive oil and put in onion and celery. Saute for 5 minutes or until fragrant and softened. Then, add cumin, paprika, garlic and chillies and stir until fragrant.

3. In a large pot, add some water, onion mixture, boiled beans, tomatoes and corn. Bring to a boil for about 15 minutes then serve in a bowl with some coriander on top.

Health fact

✓ Black beans are good to reduce constipation and bloating as it is rich in fibre. However, it is high in calorie (218 calories per 100 grams) and should be taken in a moderate amount. Moreover, the magnesium content in black beans helps to improve bone health as it plays a crucial role in various metabolism activities in the body.

✓ Asian cuisines are typically served with rice, making it a complete meal. A complete meal means all nutrients are present, and it is only a matter of the amount of salt and oil as well as the overall ingredients being put into the dishes. A complete meal sounds healthy but there are many things that should be given the attention to if you're really looking to eat healthy.

LUNCH

Lunch is an important meal for those who would like lose weight. Some individuals may think that it is okay to skip lunch and that skipping lunch could make them lose weight faster, thus growing a habit of skipping lunch. Some are even confused as to why they're not losing much weight when they have "eaten less" throughout the day. Therefore, plant-based lunches are useful for these types of individuals who would rather go hungry than filling themselves up by eating healthy foods packed with nutrients. If you don't prefer to eat heavy for lunch, then you may find some light snack in the salad and soups section of this book. Otherwise, the following list of recipes might put you to interest and break your habit of skipping lunch.

1. Stuffed bell peppers with tofu and zucchini
2. Tasty greens with garlic
3. Spiral pasta with tofu, zucchini and bell peppers
4. Zucchini noodles with portobello bolognaise
5. Sweet and sour cauliflower with rice
6. Simple cauliflower rice
7. Mushroom, kale and barley pilaf
8. Tofu tacos
9. Middle eastern style plant-based pizza

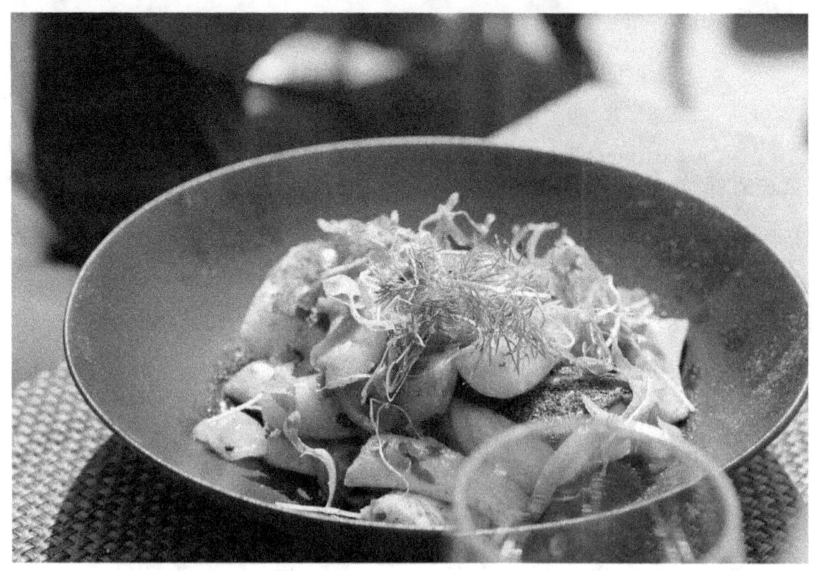

STUFFED BELL PEPPERS WITH TOFU AND ZUCCHINI

Ingredients:

- 2 bell peppers, halved

- 1 block of firm tofu, drained and cut into small cubes

- 1 zucchini, chopped into small cubes

- 1 clove garlic, minced

- 2 cups plain water

- ¼ red onion, finely chopped

- ¼ cup tomato sauce

- ½ cup spinach

- 1 tsp oregano

- 1 tsp basil

- Olive oil

- Salt and pepper

Methods:

1. Fill in a medium pot with plain water then put in the bell peppers. Bring to a boil for 10 minutes or until the peppers are soft and tender, then drain the water out.

2. In a skillet or a non-stick pan, heat some olive oil to be used to saute the onion until softened or golden brown. Then add

in the tofu and zucchini, saute again until they are brownish in colour, then add in the garlic and cook until golden brown.

3. Next, add in tomato sauce, oregano, basil and spinach until the spinach is slightly wilted. Put in salt and pepper as well to taste. Set aside and leave to cool.

4. After the tofu mixture has been cooled off, stuff the bell peppers with the mixture and serve on a plate.

Health fact

✓ Tomato sauce is a good alternative to cream-based sauces as it contains lower calorie which is about 100 calories for one cup. It is also fat-free and thus great for a low-fat diet.

✓ Basil have anti-aging properties which could prevent wrinkles, thus is good for the skin health.

TASTY GREENS WITH GARLIC

Ingredients:

- 20 stalks kale, torn

- 3 cloves garlic, minced

- ½ tbsp parsley, minced

- ¼ cup cherry tomatoes, halved

- 2 cups plain water

- 1 tbsp almond, roughly chopped (optional)

- Olive oil

- Salt and pepper

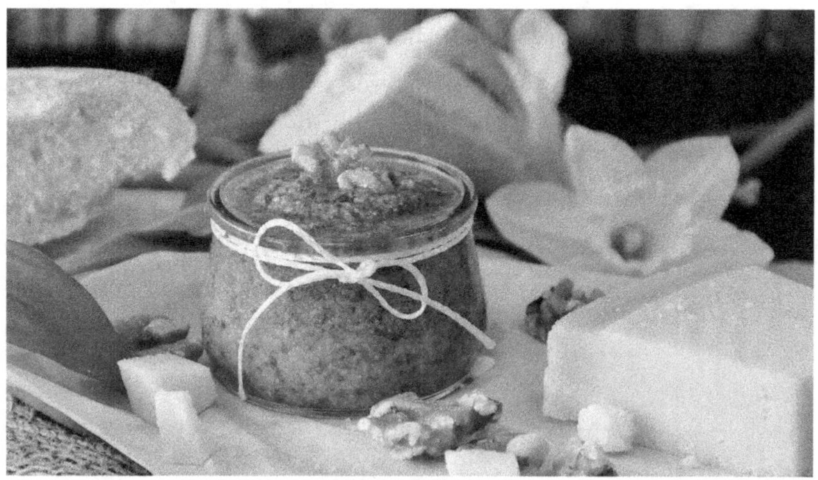

TASTY GREENS WITH GARLIC

Methods:

5. In a medium pot, boil the kale with some water, enough to cover the surface until soft and tender. Remove with a small hand-held strainer and throw the remaining water.

6. Heat some oil in the same pot used for boiling, over a medium heat. Then add in tomatoes and garlic, saute for 30 seconds. Next, add in the kale, parsley and some salt and pepper to taste. Serve in a salad bowl. Sprinkle some almond if you prefer to have some crunchiness in your bite.

Health fact

✓ Kale is said to be the healthiest food on the planet with only 33 calories, according to the Healthline. Surprisingly, kale contains way more vitamin C than oranges per cup, which are known to be beneficial for the skin.

✓ Citrus fruits are rich in health benefits such as protecting against diseases and assisting in digestion. Citrus fruits are commonly sour in taste and that they usually being turned into juices. However, fruit juices contain more sugars and should be avoided. The sugar content in fruit juices are the same as soda. Therefore, always opt for whole fruits if you want to stay on the right track of eating healthy diet.

SPIRAL PASTA WITH TOFU, ZUCCHINI AND BELL PEPPERS

Ingredients:

- 2 cups spiral pasta, cooked

- ½ block of tofu, thinly sliced

- ½ zucchini, thinly sliced

- 1 bell pepper, halved

- ¼ tbsp thyme

- ½ red onion, thinly sliced

- 2 cloves garlic, chopped

- 1 tbsp chilli paste

- Corn oil (for frying the tofu)

- Olive oil

- Salt and pepper

Methods:

1. In a large pan, pour about 3 cups of corn oil and then add in the thinly sliced tofu. Deep fry until golden brown and crispy on the outside. Set aside.

2. In another pan, heat some olive oil and then put in onion and garlic. Stir until fragrant. Add in the bell pepper, thyme, fried tofu, zucchini and chilli paste and stir until well combined

and cooked. Put some salt and pepper to taste and finally toss them together with the pasta in a large bowl. Drizzle some olive oil and ready to be served.

Health fact

- ✓ Thyme have been used to treat symptoms such as diarrhoea, sore throat and stomach-ache. Typically, it comes in two forms; essential oil and dried leaves for cooking. Moreover, the essential oil infused with thyme could be used to cure skin infections which are commonly caused by fungi.

ZUCCHINI NOODLES WITH PORTOBELLO BOLOGNAISE

Ingredients:

- 5 zucchinis, thinly sliced using a spiralizer or a julienne peeler

- 3 cups portobello mushroom, thinly sliced

- 1 ½ carrot, minced

- 1 stick celery, minced

- 1 yellow onion, minced

- 2 cloves garlic, minced

- 1 tbsp tomato puree

- ½ can crushed tomatoes

- 2 tsp oregano

- Olive oil

- Salt and pepper

Methods:

1. Place your pre-made zucchini into a large bowl and toss with some salt and pepper to taste. Transfer some of those into a plate. Set aside to prepare for the other ingredients.

2. In a large pan, heat some olive oil and add in onion and garlic, stir until fragrant. Then put in the mushroom, carrot and

celery, saute until cooked and softened which is for about 10 minutes.

3. Add the tomato puree and crushed tomatoes into the mixture, as well as some oregano and salt and pepper. Stir for 30 seconds so that they are well incorporated and then leave to bubble up for about 10 minutes. Next, put a dollop of the sauce mixture on top of the zucchini and serve with your favourite drinks.

Health fact

✓ Canned tomatoes are believed to be cooked during the canning process, and that they are found to contain lycopene, a type of antioxidant which can only be absorbed by the body when a certain food is cooked. With that being said, researchers found that canned tomatoes have higher content of cancer-resistance lycopene than the normal ones. However, if you're not using the whole can of tomatoes, it is advisable that you transfer the leftovers into a jar or contained to avoid further contact with the aluminium sourced from the can itself, which may affect our health in the long run.

SWEET AND SOUR CAULIFLOWER WITH RICE

Ingredients:

- 2 cups cauliflower florets

- 1 ½ cup white rice or brown rice

- ¼ cup corn starch

- ¼ tbsp ketchup

- 2 tbsp soy sauce

- 1 stick spring onion (for garnish)

- Sesame seed

- Olive oil

- Corn oil (to fry the cauliflower florets)

- Salt and pepper

- Water (to cook rice)

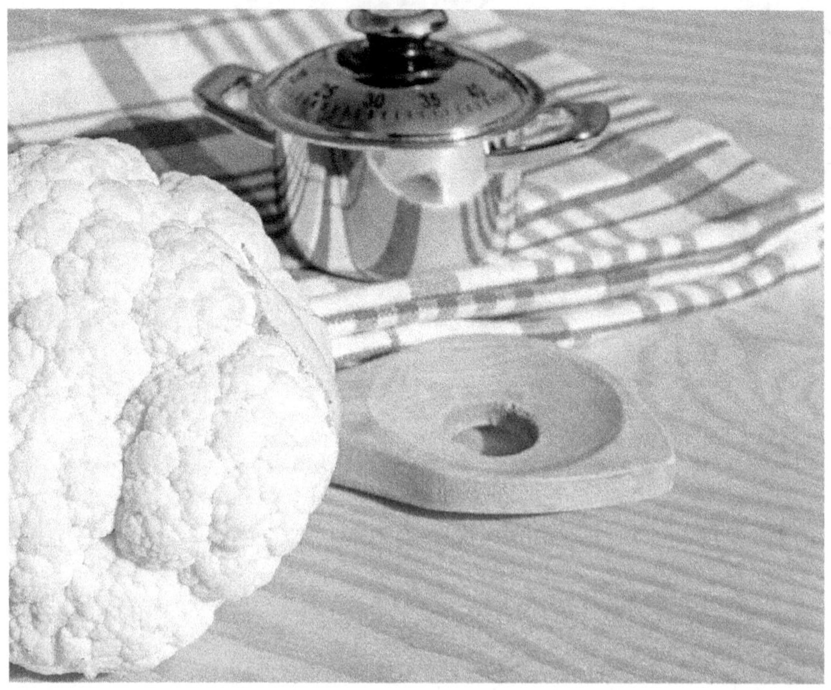

Methods:

1. To cook the rice, place the rice into your rice cooker pot and put in some water enough to cover your palm on top of the rice. Cook the rice as per your rice cooker instruction.

2. In a medium bowl, toss the cauliflower florets with the corn starch and some salt and pepper. Heat a large pan with 3 cups of corn oil and then insert the already mixed florets. Deep fry until golden brown and crispy on the outside. Drain the excess oil and transfer into a medium bowl. Set aside to prepare for the sauce.

3. For the sauce, mix in the ketchup, soy sauce, some salt and pepper, and sesame seed in a small bowl. Then pour over the fried florets, toss until well-combined. Garnish by sprinkling some spring onion on top.

4. Serve with a bowl of hot rice and enjoy your lunch.

Health fact

- ✓ This sweet and sour cauliflower is great as a replacement to the sweet and sour chicken, especially for those who craves for the latter menu. It has a complete set of nutrients; carbohydrates, proteins, fat, vitamins and minerals, all fit in one dish.

- ✓ Brown rice is much healthier than white rice because it is made up of whole grain containing bran and germ, which are removed from the white rice during the process.

SIMPLE CAULIFLOWER RICE

Ingredients:

- 1 medium-sized head of cauliflower

- 1 tbsp olive oil

- Salt and pepper

- Soy sauce (optional)

Methods:

5. Wash the cauliflower thoroughly and then separate the florets into pieces.

1. To turn your cauliflower florets into a rice form, you can either grate them using the cheese grater or using the food processor. However, if you're using a food processor, cut the hard part of the florets. Remove any excess moisture by using a paper towel or a dry cloth to ensure that your rice is not soggy.

2. In a large skillet or pan with heated olive oil, simply saute your rice and season with salt and pepper. Cook for about 8 minutes or until it is soft and tender. You may also add soy sauce to add extra taste to it.

3. Serve in a plat and you're ready to dig in!

Health fact

- ✓ Cauliflower rice can be eaten cooked or raw, depending on your preference. It is also suitable for an alternative fried rice, just like how you usually cook with white or brown rice. Furthermore, it is obvious by now that cauliflower rice is the healthiest rice and have the lowest calorie compared to the normal grains.

MUSHROOM, KALE AND BARLEY PILAF

Ingredients:

- ½ cup button mushroom, thinly sliced
- ½ leek, trimmed and sliced
- ½ cup barley, rinsed
- ½ cup kale, trimmed and chopped
- ½ stick celery, chopped
- 2 cloves garlic, minced
- 1 tbsp walnuts, chopped
- ½ cup plain water
- ½ cup vegetable broth
- 2 tbsp extra virgin olive oil
- Salt and pepper

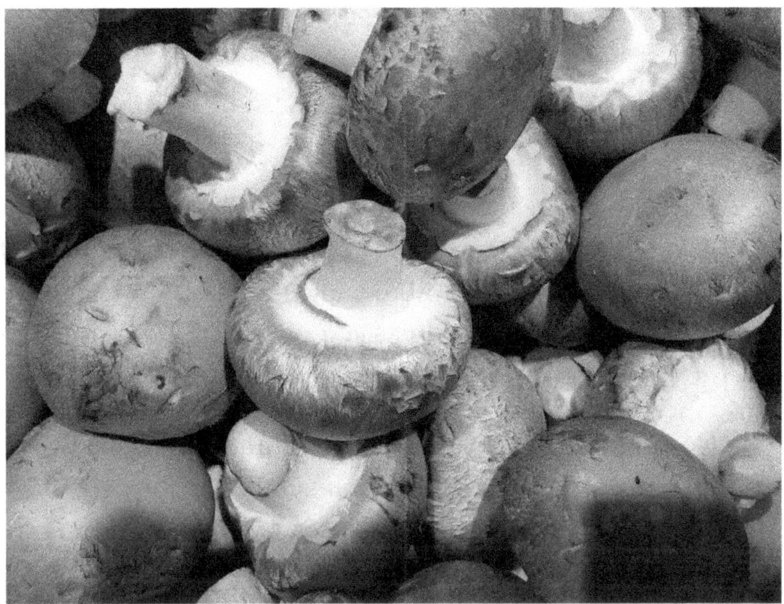

Methods:

1. Preheat the oven to 180 degree Celsius.

2. Heat olive oil in a skillet or a pan over a medium heat then add leek and celery. Saute until cooked or softened, then add in garlic.

3. Put in the barley, vegetable broth and water and bring to a boil. Then lower the heat to bring to a simmer for about 30 minutes, until the barley has absorbed the broth.

4. While the broth is simmering, spray a baking tray with some vegetable oil and spread the mushroom evenly. Roast for about 20 minutes or until golden brown.

5. Add in the roasted mushroom and some kale into the barley broth mixture and stir until kale has wilted. Put in some salt and pepper to taste. Serve in a plate and top with walnuts for a crunchy taste.

Health fact

- ✓ Barley is rich in fibre and helps to resist hunger and reduce weight. It is suitable for individuals who are afraid of having lunch due to a concern that they might gain weight. Furthermore, the high fibre content in barley could prevent gallstones which could cause a painful effect if it is stuck in your duct.

- ✓ Cooking mushrooms will not lower their nutritional values. In fact, most mushrooms sustained the nutrition even while cooking.

TOFU TACOS

Ingredients:

- 1 sheet taco shells, roasted

- 1 block tofu, cubed into bite-sized pieces

- 2 cloves garlic, finely chopped

- ½ tomato, cubed into bite-sized pieces

- ½ yellow onion, finely chopped

- ½ tsp chilli powder

- ½ tsp paprika

- ½ tbsp tomato sauce

- Olive oil

- Salt and pepper

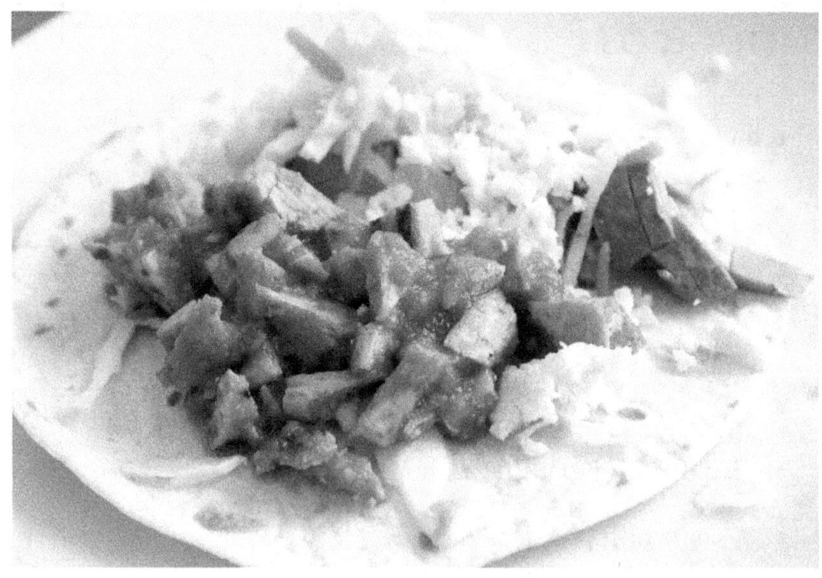

Methods:

1. In a skillet or non-stick pan, heat some olive oil and put in tofu, garlic and onion. Saute until cooked. Then add in the tomato, chilli powder, paprika, tomato sauce, and salt and pepper. Stir for 3 minutes and turn off the heat.

2. Put 2-3 spoonful of the filling on a taco shell then fold over. Enjoy your taco with your favourite wine!

Health fact

✓ Taco shells are generally gluten free since they are made up of corn and water. It is safe for individuals with wheat allergies to enjoy a filling and tasty meal just like other normal persons without having to worry about the ingredients.

✓ Paprika contains carotenoids which are often linked to hair strength.

MIDDLE EASTERN STYLE PLANT-BASED PIZZA

Ingredients:

- 1 naan bread

- ½ small-sized tomato, thinly sliced

- ½ cup tofu, thinly sliced into bite pieces and fried

- 2 cloves garlic, minced

- 1 tsp paprika

- 1 tsp cumin

- 1 tsp chilli flakes

- 1 tsp tomato paste

- Olive oil

- Salt and pepper

Methods:

1. Preheat the oven to 180 degree Celsius.

2. In a skillet or pan, heat some olive oil and stir in garlic, paprika, cumin until cooked and well combined. Then add in the tomato paste, chilli flakes, salt and pepper, stir well. Set aside to cool.

3. Spread the pizza base on top of the naan bread, then line up some fried tofu and tomatoes on top. Put it in the oven and

bake for about 5-8 minutes until the bread is crispy and golden brown. Cut into slices using a pizza cutter or a knife.

4. Serve and enjoy your meal.

Health fact

✓ Naan bread consists of 247 calories. However, despite being high in calorie, it is still considered as healthy because it is only made up of salt, whole wheat flour and water. The high calorie content could give you some energy to face the day.

✓ 1 slice of pizza contains about 280 calories which makes it a thousand calories when a whole pizza is consumed!

DINNER

Dinner is one of the important components for a complete, healthy diet. Generally, people are recommended to eat dinner at least 4 hours before bedtime to ensure that the body system digests all of the food before going to sleep. Moreover, researchers found out that eating dinner earlier could lead to a slimmer figure. This is because when you eat earlier, it gives you a better and deep sleep without having to feel hungry in the middle of the night which will eventually lead you to find food or snacks. Eating late at night will only store the food as fats in your body and in turn would make you gain some weight. However, this fact isn't entirely true because it also depends on what you eat at night. For example, it's better to look for healthy and low-calorie snacks such as salad instead of looking for high-calorie fast food like burgers and fries. In the following list of recipes are some suggestions to add to your list of plant-based dinner meals. However, you can refer to the previous salad and soup sections if you prefer to have a light dinner.

1. Vegetarian meatballs with spaghetti
2. Lentil Shepherd's pie
3. Creamy chowder with corn and fennel
4. Tofu kebabs with zucchini and eggplants
5. Korean style tofu
6. Turmeric cauliflower
7. Spicy stir-fry tofu

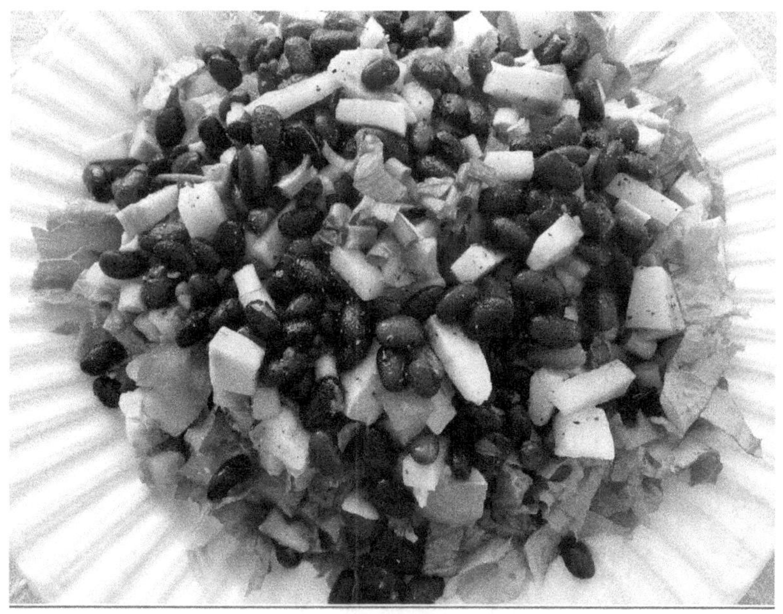

VEGETARIAN MEATBALLS WITH SPAGHETTI

Ingredients:

Meatballs:

- 3 cups fermented soybean

- 2 cloves garlic, minced

- ½ yellow onion, minced

- ¼ tbsp corn flour

- ¼ tsp oregano

- ¼ tsp basil

- ¼ cup wholemeal breadcrumb

- Water

- Olive oil

- Salt and pepper

Spaghetti sauce:

- 1 cup spaghetti, cooked

- 2 canned mashed tomatoes

- ½ yellow onion, minced

- 1 clove garlic, minced

- Olive oil

- Salt and pepper

Methods:

For the meatballs:

1. Preheat the oven to 250 degree Celsius.

2. In a skillet or a non-stick pan, saute garlic and onion until fragrant. Set aside.

3. Put the fermented soybean into a food processor and blend to break down the blocks. Then add in the onion and garlic mixture, oregano, basil, corn flour and some salt and pepper. Gradually add water while mixing, but don't let the mixture to be too runny or too sticky. Take out the mixtures then form some balls, resembling the actual meatballs.

4. In a medium bowl, cover the balls in the breadcrumb. Line a baking tray with a baking sheet and place the breadcrumb-covered meatballs then put in the oven for baking for about 15-20 minutes until golden brown.

For the sauce:

1. Over a medium heat, sautee the onion and garlic with a heated olive oil in a skillet until cooked. Then add the mashed tomatoes with some salt and pepper to taste. Leave to boil over a low heat.

Spaghetti preparation:

1. Place the cooked spaghetti in a medium plate then top with the sauce and baked meatballs.

2. Serve with your favourite drinks, best eaten when it's still warm.

Health fact

- ✓ Vegetarian meatballs contain slightly lower calorie than the actual meatballs with about 100 calories per 3 meatballs compared to 160 calories per 4 meatballs for the latter version. This make it a great alternative for plant-based diet eaters.

LENTIL'S SHEPHERD'S PIE

Ingredients:

- 1 ½ cups brown or green lentils, uncooked (rinsed and drained)

- 2 cloves garlic, minced

- ½ yellow onion, diced

- 3 cups vegetable broth

- 5 medium-sized potatoes, boiled and roughly cut into small pieces

- 1 tsp thyme

- 1 ½ cups frozen mixed veggies, thawed (diced carrots, corn, peas)

- Chopped parsley (for garnish)

- Olive oil

- Salt and pepper

Methods:

1. Preheat oven to 220 degree Celsius and prepare a baking tray sprayed with vegetable oil.

2. In a saucepan, heat some olive oil and then saute the garlic and onion until cooked and fragrant. Then add the broth, lentils, thyme, mixed veges, salt and pepper and bring to a

boil. Reduce the heat and simmer for about 35 minutes until the lentils are softened.

3. Meanwhile, put the potatoes into a large bowl and mashed them with a fork until smooth. Add some salt and pepper for seasoning.

4. Next, add about 2-3 tbsp of mashed potatoes into the broth mixtures to get a thick consistency. Transfer the mixture into an already prepared baking tray and top with the rest of the mashed potatoes. Spread evenly. Place the tray into the oven then bake for 20 minutes or until the surface is brownish in colour.

5. Before serving, let cool and garnish with some chopped parsley.

Health fact

✓   Soaking lentils for too long in water will make it lose some of its nutritional value. The best way to cook lentils is by boiling them for about 5-20 minutes. Moreover, lentils can be cooked right away instead of having to soak them first, unlike other legumes.

CREAMY CHOWDER WITH CORN AND FENNEL

Ingredients:

- 1 ½ cup frozen corn, thawed

- 1 stick fennel, chopped

- 2 green chillies, chopped

- ½ yellow onion, thinly sliced

- ½ cup fresh coriander, chopped

- 1 cup almond milk

- ½ cup vegetable broth

- Olive oil

- Salt and pepper

Methods:

1. Heat about 2 tbsp of olive oil in a medium pot over a medium heat. Then add onion and fennel to saute until fragrant. Then add in the corn, chillies and coriander and stir until cooked for about 10-15 minutes.

2. Next, add in the almond milk and vegetable broth and bring to a boil. When it has boiled, reduce the heat and simmer for about 15-20 minutes. Take out about ¾ cups of the mixture and put into a blender, then blend until smooth and creamy. Put it back into the pot with the unblended mixtures and stir

until well incorporated. Add salt and pepper to taste then turn off the heat, let cool for 10 minutes.

3. Serve in a medium bowl and garnish with fresh coriander on top.

Health fact

✓ Coriander could reduce the harmful cholesterol level in our body while increasing the good ones. Apart from that, it is also beneficial for diabetic patients as it could trigger the insulin production and reduce the blood sugar levels. It is also used to treat mouth ulcers.

✓ Surprisingly, frozen corns have a lower calorie value compared to the fresh ones with 60 calories to 72 calories. However, the amount of sodium in both corns are equal with 0.7 mg respectively. Carbohydrate and protein contents in frozen corns are slightly lower than that of fresh ones.

TOFU KEBABS WITH ZUCCHINI AND EGGPLANTS

Ingredients:

Vegetables

- 1 block tofu, cubed into bite-sized pieces (also drained and pressed for a few minutes to make it firm)

- 1 zucchini, cubed into bite-sized pieces

- 1 eggplant, cubed into bite-sized pieces

- 1 whole red onion, sliced about 1 cm

- Vegetable oil

Marinade

- 3 cloves garlic, minced

- 1 lemon, squeezed to get the juice

- ½ tbsp mixed herbs

- ¼ cup olive oil

- Salt and pepper

Methods:

1. Heat up the charcoal barbecue

2. Mix all the ingredients together in a bowl, take out about half of the marinade mixture and place in another bowl. Marinade

the tofu in one bowl while the vegetables in the other bowl. Let sit to absorb the juices for about 15-20 minutes.

3. Thread the tofu and vegetables onto skewers and grill for about 15 minutes until golden brown. Turn over the kebabs every now and then while grilling to ensure an even cooking.

4. Serve with rice or pasta or might as well eat as it is.

Health fact

✓ Vegetable oil is more suitable to be used for grilling compared to olive oil due to its high smoking point, which means that it doesn't burn as easily as olive oil. Olive oil has low smoking point in general, and that when it is heated on a high heat, it could become carcinogenic which is harmful to the body.

✓ Eggplants are very low in calorie, with only 82 calories per cup. However, eggplants contain high antioxidant substances which could shield against damages to our cells.

KOREAN STYLE TOFU

Ingredients:

- 1 block tofu, cubed into bite-sized pieces (drained and pressed in paper towels for 30 minutes)

- 2 cloves garlic, minced

- 5 tbsp soy sauce

- 2 tbsp maple syrup

- ¼ chilli flakes

- 1 tsp sesame seeds

- 1 tsp fresh ginger, grated

- Spring onion, finely chopped (for garnish)

- Olive oil

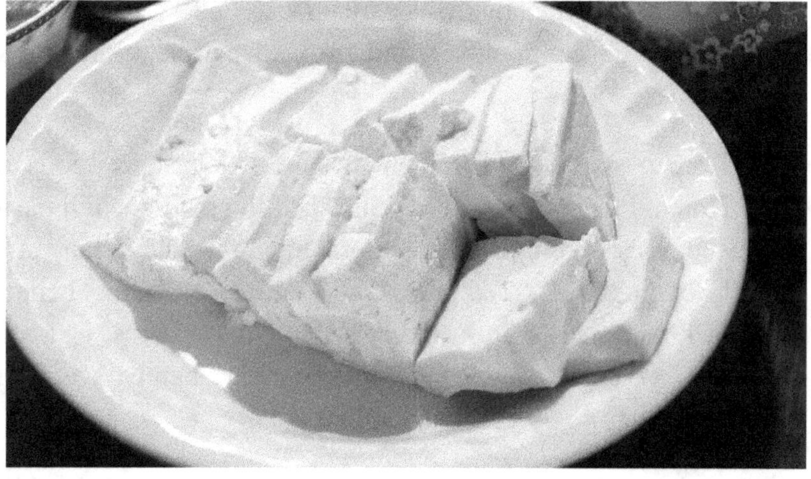

Methods:

5. In a bowl, mix together the garlic, maple syrup, chilli flakes and ginger until well combined. Put in soy sauce and let it simmer over a low heat for about 10 minutes. Next, add in firm tofu into the mixture and carefully toss them until well coated. Set aside for 30 minutes to let it absorb the soy sauce mixture.

6. After 30 minutes, heat some olive oil in a skillet or a non-stick pan over a medium heat. Then put in the tofu mixed in soy sauce and stir gently. Flip over the tofu as one side is cooked then remove from heat.

7. Serve with rice with some sesame seeds and spring onion on top as garnish.

Health fact

✓ Spring onions are rich in vitamin A, C and calcium. It could lower the risk of heart attacks and strokes. Spring onions are commonly found in the Japanese, Korean and Chinese food.

✓ Korean staple food, kimchi is one of the super foods in Korea. It is made up of cabbages, chilli powder, chilli paste and other ingredients and is fermented for a period of time. The longer it is, the better. One of the most distinct benefit of kimchi is that it decelerates the aging process, which is why you could see that most Koreans barely age even when they're 50 years and above.

TURMERIC CAULIFLOWER

Ingredients:

- 3 cups cauliflower florets

- 2 cloves garlic, minced

- 1 tsp ground turmeric

- ¼ tsp ground cumin

- 1 tsp lemon juice

- 2 ½ tbsp extra virgin olive oil

- Salt and pepper

Methods:

1. Preheat the oven to 220 degree Celsius.

2. In a medium bowl, put in the garlic, ground turmeric, ground cumin, oil, salt and pepper. Mix together until well incorporated. Then add in the cauliflower florets, toss until evenly coated with the oil mixture.

3. Spray a baking tray with vegetable oil and evenly spread the mixed cauliflower florets in the tray. Bake for about 20 minutes until it turns golden brown. Drizzle some lemon juice for a tangy taste. Serve with rice.

Health fact

- ✓ Turmeric could boost the brain functionalities and reduce brain-related diseases. Furthermore, it could also help to avoid and treat cancer.

- ✓ Cumin provides many benefits to our health, as much as other spices. Some of the benefits including for producing breast milk for breastfeeding mothers, assist in digestion, cure memory loss, acts as a natural laxative which is good for constipation and sustain healthy skin.

SPICY STIR FRY TOFU

Ingredients:

- 2 ½ blocks tofu, cubed into bite-sized pieces

- ½ green bell pepper, sliced

- ½ red bell pepper, sliced

- ½ cup bean sprouts

- ½ yellow onion, thinly sliced

- ¼ cup plain water

- 3 chillies, chopped

- 1 tsp corn starch

- Olive oil

- Salt and pepper

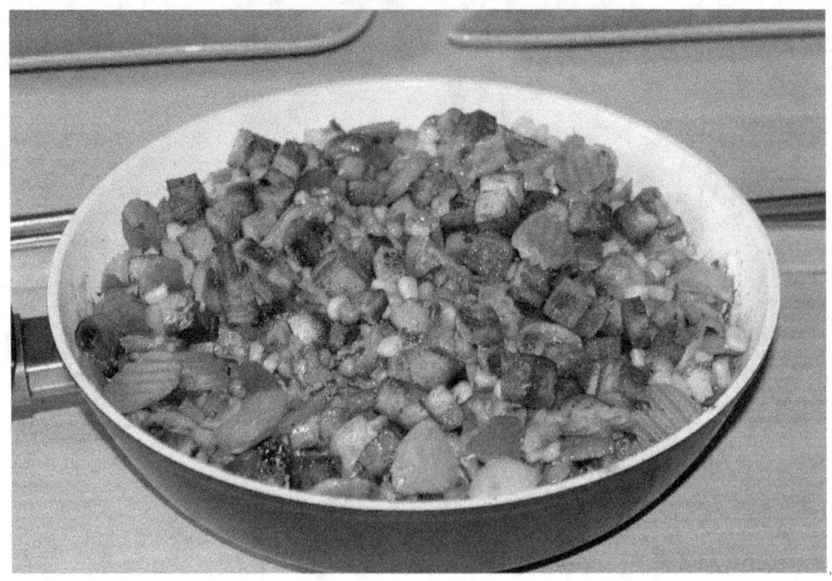

Methods:

1. In a wok, heat some olive oil over a medium-high heat. Add in the onion, bean sprouts, bell peppers, chillies and stir until fragrant and tender.

2. Next, add in some tofu and water. Simmer for about 5 minutes over the same heat then add in corn starch so that it's not too watery. Stir the tofu gently until cooked then add salt and pepper for seasoning.

3. Serve with warm rice.

Health fact

✓ Chillies are famously known for its benefit of weight reduction. This is due to the nature of this vegetable which produce heat to the eaters, which consumes their energy and thus, calories.

✓ Stir-frying or sautéing your vegetables is much better than steaming them because you could still retain the nutrients by stir-frying or sautéing. Steaming your vegetables would only make your vegetables lose the nutrients and colouration through the steam.

DESSERTS/SNACKS

A one-day meal won't be complete without desserts. Many people think that plant-based desserts never existed as the foods in this group are often associated as unhealthy, high-calorie and high sugar content. Well this is absolutely untrue! Plant-based diet eaters could still enjoy delicious desserts after consuming the so-called plain and too nutritious foods (according to non-plant-based diet eaters). As you may have noticed now, there are plenty of substitutes that could be used in desserts as well. With food, there are many possibilities and trial and error that everyone could experiment. It is a matter of how we perceive things and apply them into our daily lives. The following list of recipes could get you thinking that it's impossible to make them by using only plant-based ingredients.

1. Grilled peaches
2. Vanilla ice cream
3. Chocolate peanut butter truffles
4. Chocolate orange mousse
5. Coconut-banana cookie
6. Pumpkin pie
7. Almond cheesecake
8. Lemon meringue pie
9. Apple pie
10. Chocolate-dipped fruits with spices
11. Mango and coconut sorbet
12. Fruity shaved ice
13. Black sesame soymilk-shake
14. Berry almond crisp
15. Almond sriracha
16. Creamy spinach

17. <u>Chocolate covered banana ice cream bars</u>

153

154

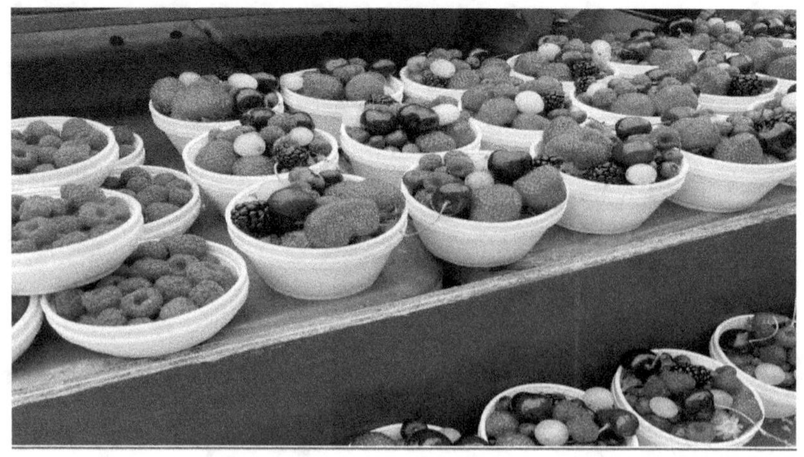

GRILLED PEACHES

Ingredients:

- 1 peach fruit, halved and removed its seed

- Plant-based ice cream or yogurt, or other cold desserts

- Olive oil

Methods:

1. Brush each side of the pair of peach with olive oil.

2. Heat the griller for about 5 minutes, then put oiled peaches on top. Grill until the marks could be seen, which is for about 5 minutes on each side.

3. Remove from heat and serve in a bowl along with 2 scoops of vanilla ice cream. Best eaten with cold desserts such as plant-based ice cream or Greek yogurt.

<u>Health fact</u>

- ✓ 150 grams of peaches contains only about 58 calories but is rich in nutrients good for fighting against diseases and as antioxidants, which are beneficial to prevent aging.

- ✓ Plant-based yogurt is also known as the Greek yogurt and they consist of coconut cream and pea protein. It contains only 59 calories per 100 grams of serving with absolutely zero fat.

VANILLA ICE CREAM

Ingredients:

- 1 ½ cups coconut milk

- ½ cup maple syrup

- 1 vanilla beans

- 1 tsp pure vanilla extract

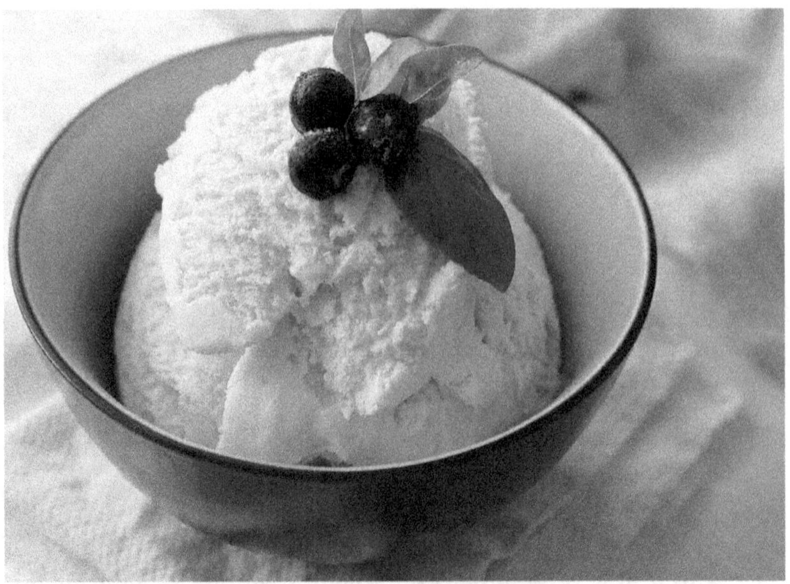

Methods:

1. Freeze your ice cream maker bowl in the freezer overnight.

2. Put all ingredients in a blender or a food processor, then blend until smooth and well incorporated. To get the vanilla beans, lay the vanilla pod on a flat surface and cut the middle with a knife, then scrap the beans out and mix with the other

ingredients. Put the mixtures into the fridge overnight to prevent crystallization process from occurring.

3. On the day after, pour the mixture into the ice cream maker bowl and turn it on to start the churning process and leave for about 25 minutes until you get a soft serve consistency.

4. Next, put the churned ice cream into an airtight container and keep it in the freezer for at least 2 hours for it to set. Highly recommended to serve it in a bowl with your favourite fruits!

Health fact

✓ Vanilla is a commonly used ingredient in desserts. One of the health benefits of vanilla is that it can be used to cure tooth decay. Other than that, its soft fragrant could also aid in boosting your mood, as well as reducing anxiety.

✓ If you're looking for plant-based ice creams at the supermarket, look for the vegan ice cream labels as vegans and plant-based are not much difference. The only difference is that vegan food are prohibited to be included with meat, dairy or eggs at all, while plant-based avoid those 3 distinctive ingredients while still having the possibility of being included.

CHOCOLATE PEANUT BUTTER TRUFFLES

Ingredients:

- 5 tbsp crunchy, unsweetened and natural peanut butter

- 2 cups dark chocolate, roughly cut into pieces

- 1 cup plant-based butter

- ½ tsp vanilla extract

- ½ tsp maple syrup

- Salt

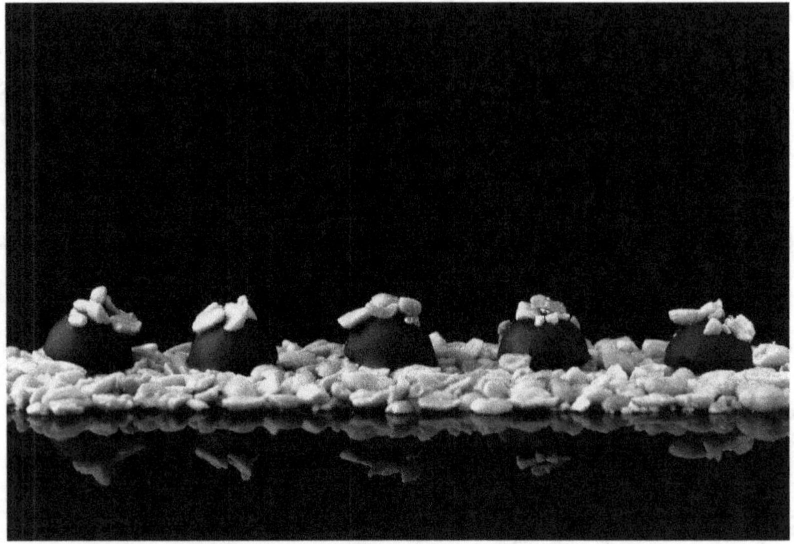

Methods:

1. In a large bowl, beat the butter by using a hand-held mixer or any mixer that you have at home, until smooth. Then add in the peanut butter, vanilla, maple syrup and salt then mix again until well combined and smooth.

2. Line a baking tin with a parchment paper. Roll the dough into balls and align them onto the baking tin. Place it in the fridge to set, for about 45 minutes to 1 hour.

3. Place the chocolate pieces into a medium bowl then microwave it in the oven for about 3 minutes until it melts. Stir the remaining clumpy chocolates until smooth.

4. Dip the peanut butter balls into the melted chocolate and place them in a fridge to set. This dessert could last for months when being kept in the fridge. But, I'm pretty sure it'd disappear within a day because it's just so addictive!

<u>Health fact</u>

✓ Dark chocolate provides more benefits that milk chocolate due to its natural form. Some of the benefits are that it could boost your brain functionalities by improving the blood flow, could lower the risk of heart diseases and lower the harmful cholesterol levels in the body, or also known as the LDL cholesterol.

CHOCOLATE ORANGE MOUSSE

Ingredients:

- 1 cup dark chocolate, roughly cut into pieces

- ½ cup orange juice

- 2 tbsp maple syrup

- 1 tsp vanilla extract

- ½ avocado

- ½ orange skin, still intact (optional)

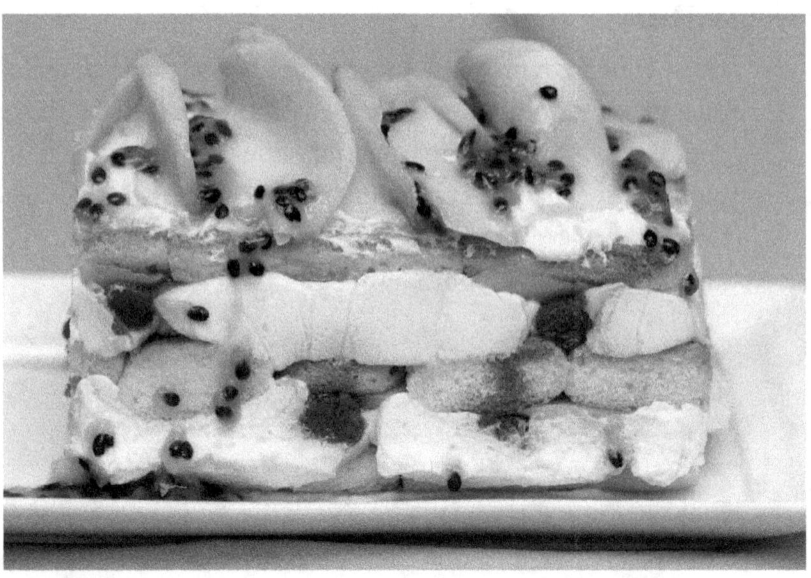

Methods:

1. Melt the chocolate using the double-boiler method or heat them in the microwave for about 3 minutes. If you're using the microwave to melt the chocolate, ensure that you stir any

leftover chunks and stir the melted the chocolate until smooth. Set aside to cool.

2. Put in the avocado in a blender or a food processor and blend until smooth. Then add in the orange juice, maple syrup and vanilla extract. You can either combine them using a spatula or blend again.

3. Scoop out the mousse into the inner part of the orange skin as decoration. Or, you could also serve them in a small bowl and enjoy your dessert.

Health fact

✓ Oranges are good source of vitamin C and good for the maintenance of your skin. However, you should not eat oranges everyday as it might interrupt your digestive system by causing diarrhoea and other fatal digestive symptoms.

✓ However, the less commonly known benefit of oranges is that it could reduce the risk of ischemic stroke among women. Ischemic stroke is when there is a blockage in the artery of your brain.

COCONUT BANANA COOKIES

Ingredients:

- 3 cups unsweetened coconut flakes

- 3 bananas, mashed

- 2 tbsp cocoa powder

- ½ tsp vanilla extract

- Salt

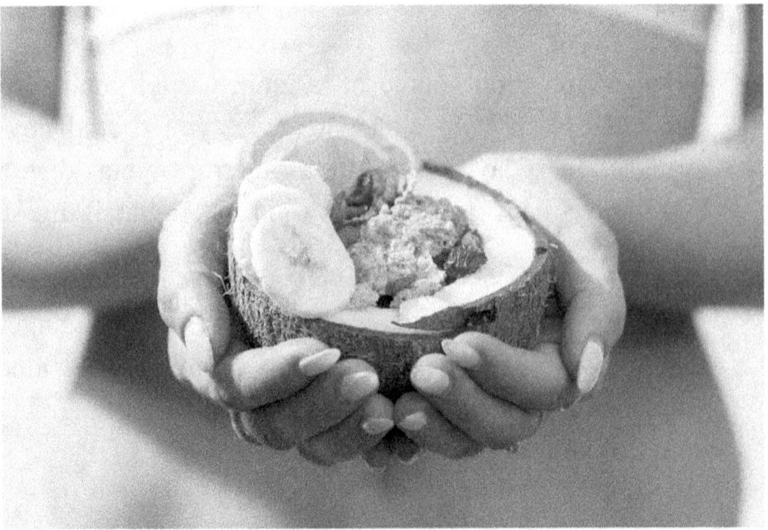

Methods:

1. Preheat the oven for 180 degree Celsius.

2. In a large bowl, mashed the bananas then add in the coconut flakes and vanilla extract. Fold over until well combined and fold again with the coconut powder. Sprinkle a pinch of salt.

3. Prepare a baking tray and line with a parchment paper or spray with vegetable oil. Scoop out the cookie dough and align accordingly. Bake for about 25 minutes or until it doesn't stick to the bottom of the paper/tray.

4. Keep in an airtight container to last for months.

Health benefit

✓ Coconut water and coconut flakes provides a strong and healthy hair.

✓ Coconut flakes should be taken moderately because it could affect the blood artery which leads to stroke. Other than that, pregnant women in the early trimester are not advisable to consume coconut flakes because there is a high chance that harmful bacteria exist in the flakes, and in turn could lead to miscarriage.

PUMPKIN PIE

Ingredients:

Crust

- 2 tbsp plant-based milk

- 1 cup rolled oats

- ¼ cup dates, pitted and softened in hot water

- ¼ cup unsalted almond butter

Salt

Filling

- 1 cup pure pumpkin puree (without additional sugar, etc.)

- 1 tsp ground cinnamon

- 1/3 cup almond or soymilk

- ½ cup maple syrup

- 2 tsp lemon juice

- ½ tsp vanilla extract

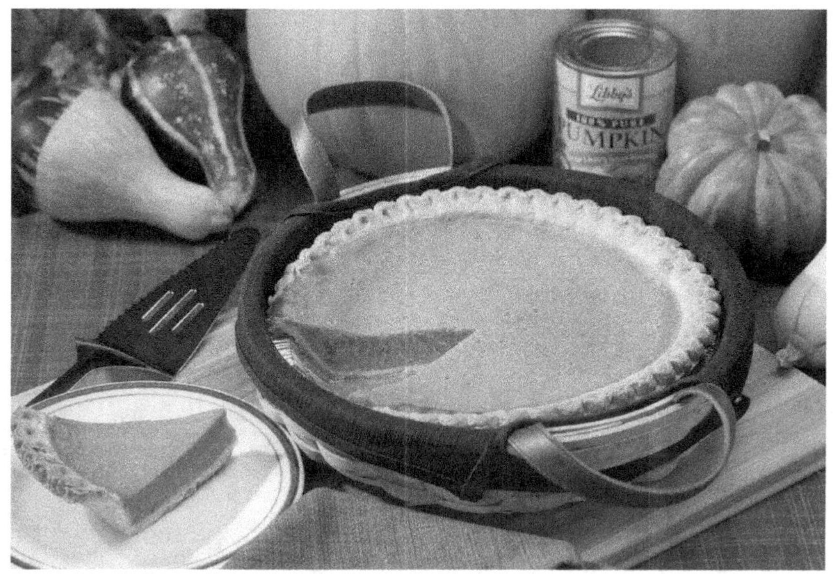

Methods:

1. Preheat the oven for 200 degree Celsius.

2. For the crust, prepare a pie plate and spray with some vegetable oil. Blend rolled oats, dates and salt in a food processor until smooth and well combined. Then add in the milk butter, blend again until solid and sticky. Evenly spread the dough into the pie plate and bake only until the edges looked cooked and crispy, then set aside to cool and prepare the filling.

3. For the filling, blend all ingredients in a blender or food processor until smooth. Then pour it into the cooled crust. Bake for about 10 minutes until the filling is set and all cooked, and the crust is completely golden brown in colour.

4. Slice your pumpkin pie and serve on a small dish. Suitable to be enjoyed during teatime, as a dessert or snack. Keep the remaining pie in an airtight container and place it in the fridge for a longer lasting crispiness of the crust.

Health fact

✓ Almond butter contains vitamin E which are good to reduce the cholesterol levels while the magnesium content in almond butter could improve the heart health.

✓ The difference with between almond butter and peanut butter is that almond butter has more nutritional content than peanut butter, thus making it a little healthier. However, peanut butter overpowered the protein content in almond butter by only a small amount.

ALMOND CHEESECAKE

Ingredients:

Cake base

- 1 ½ cup raw almonds, sliced

- 1 ½ tbsp cocoa powder

- ½ cup almond milk

- Salt

Filling

- 1 cup raw cashews, soaked and rinsed

- 2 tbsp almond butter

- ½ tbsp lemon juice

- ¼ cup maple syrup

- ½ tbsp vanilla extract

- ½ cup water

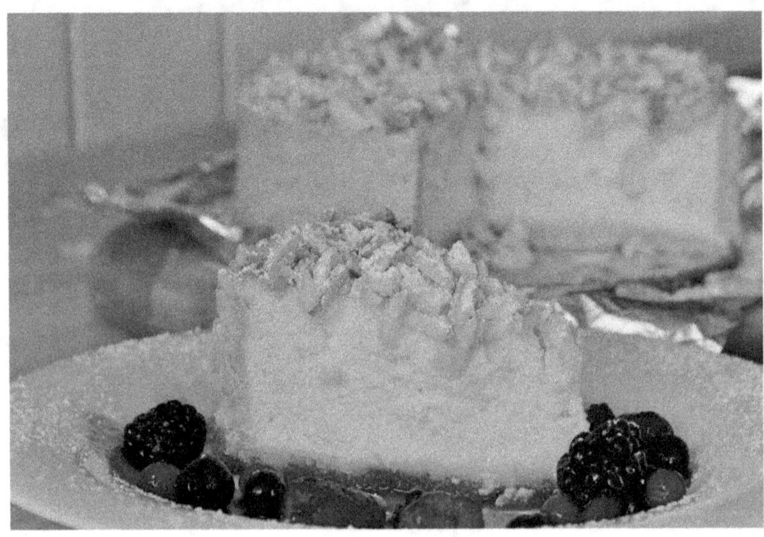

Methods:

1. For the cake base, prepare a baking tin measured 8x8 and line with a parchment paper or spray with vegetable oil. In a food processor, blend the almonds and cocoa powder until finely crushed, then add in almond milk and salt until well incorporated. Then, spread the base mixture evenly in the baking tin and set aside to prepare for the filling.

2. For the filling, blend all ingredients in a blender until smooth and creamy.

3. Add the filling into the baking tray and store it in the fridge to let it set, which is for about 30 minutes. Slice and serve with vanilla ice cream.

<u>Health fact</u>

✓ Almonds or any nuts contains an abundant amount of fibre and protein which could reduce your calorie intake. This is because nuts are good to resist hunger which in turn could help you to control your eating habit.

✓ Plant-based cheese contains quite similar nutrients to dairy cheese. One of the nutrients is commonly found in soy-based cheese called casein which is a protein similar to that found in dairy cheese. Casein is also an agent which provide a similar texture to the dairy cheese.

LEMON MERINGUE PIE

Ingredients:

Crust

- 2 tbsp plant-based milk

- 1 cup rolled oats

- ¼ cup dates, pitted and softened in hot water

- ¼ cup unsalted almond butter

- Salt

Curd

- ½ tbsp corn starch, mixed with 4 tbsp water

- 4 tbsp lemon juice (3 for the curd, 1 for the meringue)

- 1 block tofu, roughly cut into pieces and rinsed

- 2 cups chickpea liquid (for the meringue)

- ½ tbsp vanilla extract

- 5 cups plain water

- 1 pack of agar-agar (can be found in Asian stores)

- ½ tbsp maple syrup

- Salt

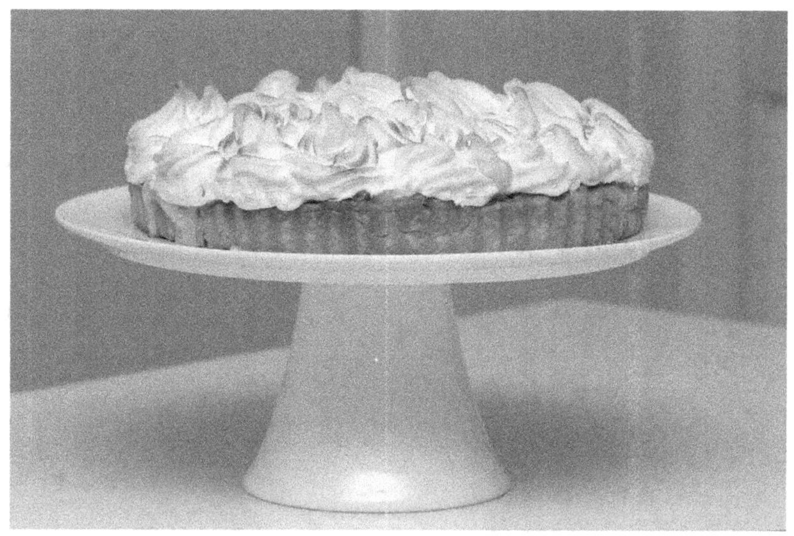

Methods:

1. Preheat the oven for 200 degree Celsius.

2. For the crust, prepare a pie plate and spray with some vegetable oil. Blend rolled oats, dates and salt in a food processor until smooth and well combined. Then add in the milk butter, blend again until solid and sticky. Evenly spread the dough into the pie plate and bake only until the edges looked cooked and crispy, then set aside to cool and prepare the curd and meringue.

3. For the curd, add in the maple syrup, lemon juice and salt. Stir until combined. Next, add in the corn starch, and stir until well mixed with the mixture. Use a medium-high heat.

4. Lower the heat to bring to a boil while keep stirring for about 5 minutes.

5. Add the mixture and tofu into a blender and blend until smooth.

6. For the meringue, use a mixer to beat the chickpea liquid and lemon juice until a stiff meringue is formed. Then add in some vanilla extract and beat again for a few seconds.

7. For the meringue syrup, boil the agar-agar in a pot of water until dissolved. Then heat up the saucepan with maple syrup. Add the maple syrup to the meringue and combine well.

8. Add the curd filling into the prepared crust and evenly top with the meringue mixtures. Let it set in the fridge for an hour to let it set. You may torch the meringue or serve as it is.

Health fact

✓ Lemon is good to freshen the breathes with its soft and tangy fragrant.

✓ Agar-agar is like a vegan version of gelatine which is often used to make jelly desserts, puddings and as soup thickening agent. Some of its health benefits are improving the digestive system and reduce the risk of anaemia.

APPLE PIE

Ingredients:

Crust

- 4 tbsp plant-based milk

- 2 cup rolled oats

- ½ cup dates, pitted and softened in hot water

- ½ cup unsalted almond butter

- Salt

Filling

- 3 apples, removed from its core and thinly sliced

- ½ tsp ground cinnamon

- ½ cup maple syrup

- ½ tbsp lemon juice

- ½ tsp ground nutmeg

- ½ cup plain flour

- ½ tbsp almond milk

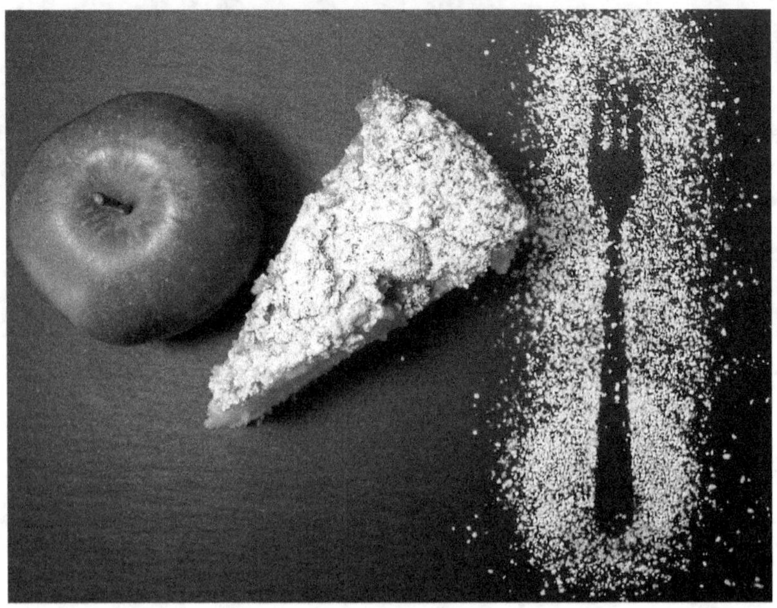

Methods:

1. Preheat the oven for 200 degree Celsius.

2. For the crust, prepare a pie plate and spray with some vegetable oil. Blend rolled oats, dates and salt in a food processor until smooth and well combined. Then add in the milk butter, blend again until solid and sticky. Evenly spread the ½ of the dough into the pie plate and bake only until the edges looked cooked and crispy, then set aside to cool and prepare the filling. Roll out the other half of the dough to cover the filling later.

3. For the filling, mix together the plain flour, ground cinnamon and ground nutmeg in a bowl. In a separate bowl, combine together the apples, lemon juice and maple syrup then add in the flour mixture.

4. Brush the crust with some almond milk then pour in the filling. Cover with the other half of the rolled dough, make small slits using a knife to let the steam out during baking. Bake for about 30 – 45 minutes. Leave to cool on a wire rack for 10 minutes.

5. Slice and serve with vanilla ice cream.

Health fact

✓ Apples are filling and that it could assist in weight loss. Apples could also shield your lungs from oxidative damage which could lead to asthma. This is due to its nature of being rich in antioxidant properties.

CHOCOLATE-DIPPED FRUITS WITH SPICES

Ingredients:

- 3 cups unsweetened dark chocolates, roughly chopped

- 2 peaches, pitted and sliced

- 4 strawberries, halved

- 1 mango, pitted and cubed

- ½ tsp ground nutmeg

- ½ tsp ground cinnamon

Methods:

1. Put the chocolate into a medium bowl and melt in a microwave for about 5 minutes. Stir the remaining chocolate chunks until smooth. Add in some ground nutmeg and cinnamon.

2. Dip in the fruits into the chocolate mixture and place in a baking tray. Put in the fridge to let it set.

3. Suitable to be served as a snack. Keep in airtight container in the fridge.

<u>Health fact</u>

✓ Fruits comes with many health benefits such as for healthy skin, reduce risk of chronic diseases, aid in weight-loss and many others. However, there is a limitation to eating fruits.

It is recommended to eat only 5 servings per day. This is because the natural sugar content in fruits might trigger the diabetes disease factor.

✓ Nutmegs are associated with sexual treatment such as increasing the sexual drive. However, this fact is applicable to animals as experiments involving human are still lacking and more research need to be done.

MANGO AND COCONUT SORBET

Ingredients:

- 2 cups mango, cubed

- ¾ cups maple syrup

- 1 tbsp lemon juice

- 1 cup coconut milk

- ¼ coconut flakes, unsweetened and toasted (for toppings)

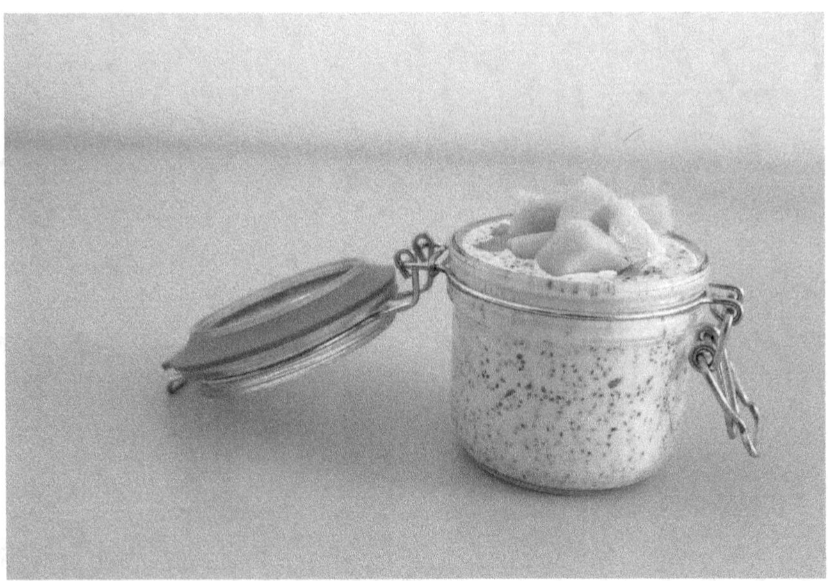

Methods:

1. Freeze an ice cream maker bowl overnight.

2. Blend in the mango, maple syrup, lemon juice and coconut milk in a blender or a food processor until smooth.

3. Place the mango mixture into the frozen ice cream maker bowl. Turn on the ice cream maker and churn until soft, for about 10 minutes.

4. Add the mixture into a container and freeze until firm. Serve in an ice cream bowl and top with some mango flakes.

Health fact

✓ One cup of mango contains 99 calories and about 70% of vitamin C. Vitamin C are good to protect our body against infections as well as for growth and repair. Other than that, mango could also improve your eye health with its vitamin A content which is often associated with night time blindness and dry eyes.

✓ Not cereals are healthy and good to be consumed daily. Those cereals that you find at the supermarkets contain more sugars than you think. Plus, you're actually consuming a lot more sugar when you add milk into your cereals. It is best to make your own breakfast bar with organic ingredients as you could control the number of calories that you put into your breakfast meal.

FRUITY SHAVED ICE

Ingredients:

- 2 cups fruit of your choice

- ½ tbsp maple syrup

- ½ tbsp lemon juice

- 1 cup water

- Ice, shaved using ice machine or blender

Methods:

1. Puree the fruit by using a blender until smooth.

2. Transfer the fruit puree into a medium saucepan, put on a medium heat and add in the lemon juice, maple syrup and water. Bring to a boil and stir the mixture every now and then. Reduce the heat then bring to a simmer for 5 minutes over the same heat. Set aside to let cool.

3. Strain the cooked and cooled puree by using a strainer to remove the seeds. Pour the syrup into a glass container and put it in the fridge to get icy cool before being poured over the shaved ice.

4. Scoop out some shaved ice into a bowl and then pour the fruit mixture over the ice until completely covered. Serve with some sliced fruits. Suitable to be serve as a dessert during the summer.

Health fact

- ✓ Consuming icy desserts like shaved ice will not lower or increase your calorie intake as ice is made up of plain water, and water does not have any calories. The only effect it could give to your health is that it could cause tooth decay or other dental problems when you munch on ice.

- ✓ Pineapples could help in providing a speedy recovery, particularly after surgeries or tissue damages caused by extreme exercises. Other than fruit, this fruit contain anti-inflammatory property which is good for our digestive system.

BLACK SESAME SOYMILK-SHAKE

Ingredients:

- 2 cups soymilk

- ½ tbsp black sesame seeds

- ½ tsp maple syrup

- ½ cup plain water

- 2 mint leaves

- 1 cup ice

Methods:

5. Combine all ingredients in a blender and blend until the ice is completely crushed. Serve in a tall glass and garnish with mint leaves.

<u>Health fact</u>

- ✓ Sesame seeds contain vitamin B which are good for metabolic processes in our body.

- ✓ Healthy milkshakes are ones that are homemade as you could control the amount or sugars or sweeteners to include in your milkshakes.

- ✓ Brown sugars are similar to the regular white sugar, but with molasses added to it which give it the brown colouration. Other than that, brown sugars contain slightly more nutrients than white sugars because of the addition of molasses. So, don't be fooled by the myth saying that brown sugars are healthier and should be used often for cooking and baking!

BERRY ALMOND CRISP

Ingredients:

- ½ cup almonds

- ½ cup rolled oats

- 4 tbsp almond butter

- 1 tbsp maple syrup

- 1 cup mixed berries of your choice

- Salt

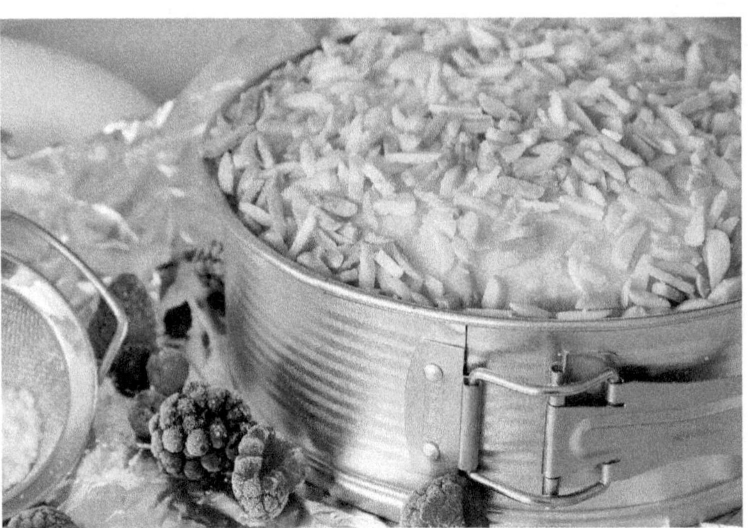

Methods:

1. Preheat the oven to 190 degree Celsius.

2. Blend the almonds and rolled oats in a food processor or a blender until they are in powdered form. Then add in the rest of the ingredients and blend until some chunks is formed.

3. Pour the mixed berries into a mini cast iron skillet and then scoop out the almond mixtures onto the berries by using a spoon. Spread evenly and bake for 20 minutes until golden brown. Serve with a scoop of vanilla ice cream.

Health fact

✓ Consuming berries could improve the mental decline especially during old age among women.

✓ Frozen berries are still packed with nutrients and freezing them will not affect their nutrient content. Furthermore, you could also keep frozen berries for months without having to worry about wasting them.

ALMOND SRIRACHA

Ingredients:

- 1 cup maple syrup

- 2 tbsp almond butter, melted

- 2 cups raw almonds

- 1 tbsp store-bought sriracha sauce

- Salt and pepper

Methods:

1. Preheat the oven to 180 degree Celsius and line a baking tray with a parchment paper or spray with some vegetable oil.

2. Combine together maple syrup, sriracha sauce, melted butter and pepper, whisk until well incorporated. Then add in the raw almonds and toss until they're covered with the mixture.

3. Pour the almond mixture into a lined baking tray and evenly spread them out. Sprinkle some salt and bake for about 15-20 minutes until crispy, stirring every now and then for an even cooking.

4. Let cool for about 10 minutes and keep it in an airtight container. Serve as a snack and best eaten when you're controlling your diet.

Health fact

- ✓ Sriracha sauce is a spicy sauce made up of chillies and garlic and is almost similar to the regular ketchup. As it is made up of chillies, it could help to lose weight due to its hot nature. Furthermore, capsaicin found in hot sauce could destroy the damaging cancer cells without affecting the healthy cells.

- ✓ According to BBC, the world's healthiest raw food is almond with a score of 97, despite having a high calorie content. Moreover, its almonds consist of all the nutrients needed by the body and it is by no surprise that it could improve our health much better than any other food available. Almonds could enhance our cardiovascular health and aid in diabetes treatment and prevention.

CREAMY SPINACH

Ingredients:

- 2 cups fresh spinach

- 1 ¼ cup plain water

- 1 cup vegetable broth

- ½ cup plant-based milk

- Salt and pepper

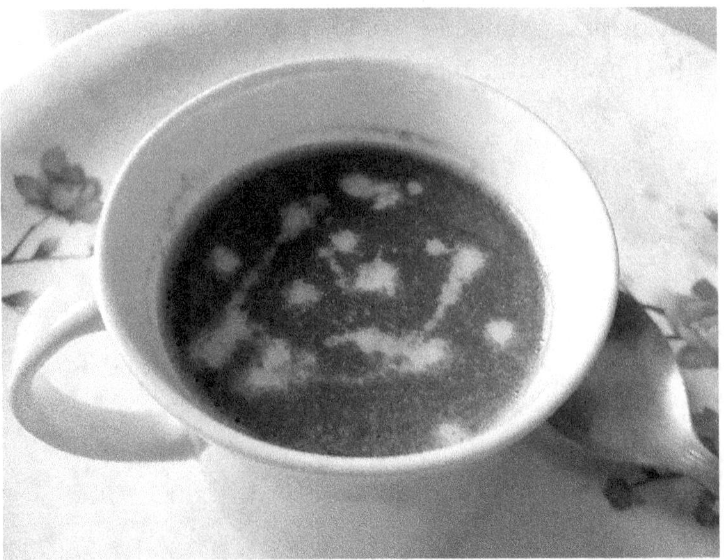

Methods:

1. Add the water into a pot and bring to a simmer for about 5 minutes over a medium-high heat. Cover with a lid to speed up the process. Then, add in the vegetable broth and stir to combine, then bring to a boil.

2. Reduce the heat and put in the fresh spinach and cook for 5 minutes. Do not let the spinach to be overcooked.

3. Further reduce the heat to low then add in the milk into the spinach mixture. Simmer for about 10 minutes. You could add more milk if you prefer a creamier texture. Add some salt and pepper to taste and serve in a bowl. Best eaten as a snack during the day.

Health fact

✓ Plant-based milk contains more ingredients than the regular dairy milk. Moreover, the regular dairy milk contains 8 times more protein compared to regular dairy milk. Plant-based milk are typically added with sugar, but you can still get the unsweetened by checking the ingredient label.

✓ Homemade vegetable broth contains less salt and zero sugars. The thing about homemade food is that you can control your salt and sugar intake in your dishes, plant-based or not. Homemade foods are also typically low in calories.

CHOCOLATE COVERED BANANA ICE CREAM BARS

Ingredients:

- 3 ½ cups dark chocolate (3 cups roughly chopped and melted, ½ cup roughly chopped)

- 2 tbsp cocoa powder

- 4 large-sized bananas, mashed

- 2 tbsp unsweetened peanut butter

Methods:

1. In a blender or food processor, add in the cocoa powder, mashed bananas and peanut butter until smooth and creamy. Add in the roughly chopped dark chocolate and fold until well-combined. Set aside to melt the rest of the chocolate chunks.

2. In a medium bowl, melt the rest of the chocolate chunks for about 4 minutes in a microwave. Stir the leftover chunks until completely melted with the rest.

3. Pour about 1 tbsp of the melted chocolate into ice cream moulds and put in the fridge to set. Ensure that there is an even coating inside the moulds.

4. When the chocolate has set, fill in the chocolate shell with the banana ice cream batter and pop with ice cream sticks. Put it in the fridge to set for about 3-4 hours.

5. Good to be served as a snack or dessert during summer. Enjoy!

Health fact

- ✓ Cocoa powder or chocolates in general is known for its benefit in improving the mood and reduce depression. This is because it contains a mood stabilizer property, triggering to pleasure of eating chocolates.

- ✓ It is recommended to consume dark chocolates with at least 70% cocoa content as it is packed with nutrients and beneficial for the health, other than ensuring that no more than that percentage of other ingredients are added into it, especially sugars.

CONCLUSION

From the recipes and facts that are provided with them, it is proven that plant-based diet mainly consists of ingredients which are generally good for the health. Moreover, most of the nutritional benefits of the ingredients used in the recipes provide similar functionalities and benefits to our health. The most common and repeated benefits are lowering the risk of cancers and provide antioxidants to the body. This would further approve the fact that plant-based diet is an ideal diet for people who would like to transition from regular diet to plant-based as it contains almost similar nutrition with the regular diet plan.

On the other hand, plant-based diet is not as complicated as you think it is and most of the ingredients are easy to get, in fact, you might even plant them at your backyard! Unlike the regular diet ingredients, in a situation where you have to find a specific animal parts, some places may run out of them and you might crave for the dish for God knows how long until the parts are available again. Meanwhile, plant-based ingredients are abundant and could be find at your nearest stores or street vendors, at a much lower cost too!

I may not be able to ask people to start eating plant-based foods, but it's good enough to make them aware of the nutrition that they consumed daily in their food plan. Furthermore, I cannot change their mind about how easy it is to cook plant-based meals, but at least they could try these recipes at home and that would make them start pondering on the coolness of practicing a plant-based diet one day.

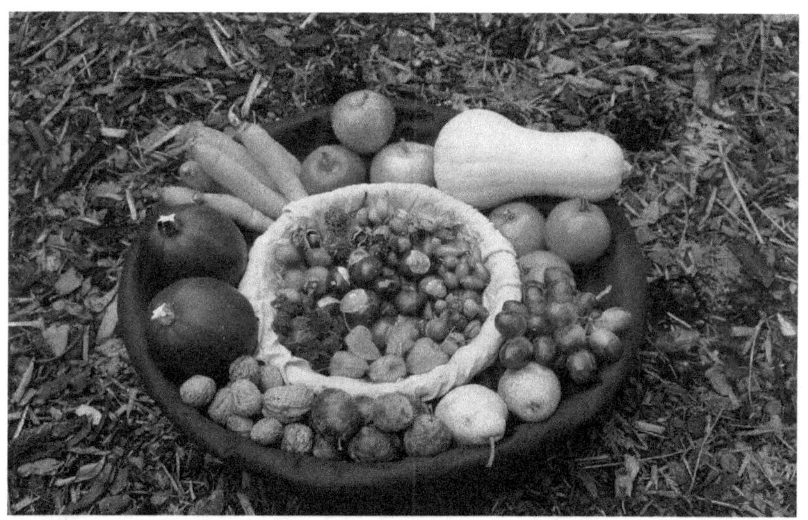

www.ingramcontent.com/pod-product-compliance
Lightning Source LLC
Chambersburg PA
CBHW070831250726
48662CB00003B/1162